Mastitis

Editors

PAMELA L. RUEGG
CHRISTINA S. PETERSSON-WOLFE

VETERINARY CLINICS OF NORTH AMERICA: FOOD ANIMAL PRACTICE

www.vetfood.theclinics.com

Consulting Editor
ROBERT A. SMITH

November 2018 • Volume 34 • Number 3

ELSEVIER

1600 John F. Kennedy Boulevard • Suite 1800 • Philadelphia, Pennsylvania, 19103-2899

http://www.vetfood.theclinics.com

VETERINARY CLINICS OF NORTH AMERICA: FOOD ANIMAL PRACTICE Volume 34, Number 3
November 2018 ISSN 0749-0720, ISBN-13: 978-0-323-64336-8

Editor: Colleen Dietzler
Developmental Editor: Meredith Madeira

Veterinary Clinics of North America: Food Animal Practice (ISSN 0749-0720) is published in March, July, and November by Elsevier Inc., 360 Park Avenue South, New York, NY 10010-1710. Subscription prices are $250.00 per year (domestic individuals), $413.00 per year (domestic institutions), $100.00 per year (domestic students/residents), $276.00 per year (Canadian individuals), $545.00 per year (Canadian institutions), $335.00 per year (international individuals), $545.00 per year (international institutions), and $165.00 per year (international and Canadian students/residents). To receive student/resident rate, orders must be accompanied by name of affiliated institution, date of term, and the signature of program/residency coordinator on institution letterhead. *Clinics* subscription prices. All prices are subject to change without notice. **POSTMASTER:** Send address changes to *Veterinary Clinics of North America: Food Animal Practice*, Elsevier Health Sciences Division, Subscription Customer Service, 3251 Riverport Lane, Maryland Heights, MO 63043. Customer Service (orders, claims, online, change of address): Elsevier Health Sciences Division, Subscription **Customer Service, 3251 Riverport Lane, Maryland Heights, MO 63043. Tel: 1-800-654-2452 (U.S. and Canada); 314-447-8871 (ouside U.S. and Canada). Fax: 314-447-8029. E-mail: journalscustomerservice-usa@elsevier.com (for print support); journalsonlinesupport-usa@elsevier.com (for online support).**

Reprints. For copies of 100 or more, of articles in this publication, please contact the Commercial Reprints Department, Elsevier Inc., 360 Park Avenue South, New York, NY 10010-1710. Tel.: 212-633-3874; Fax: 212-633-3820; E-mail: reprints@elsevier.com.

Veterinary Clinics of North America: Food Animal Practice is covered in *Current Contents/Agriculture, Biology and Environmental Sciences, MEDLINE/PubMed (Index Medicus),* and *Excerpta Medica.*

Contributors

CONSULTING EDITOR

ROBERT A. SMITH, DVM, MS
Diplomate, American Board of Veterinary Practitioners; Veterinary Research and
Consulting Services, LLC, Greeley, Colorado, USA

EDITORS

PAMELA L. RUEGG, DVM, MPVM
Professor and Chairperson, Department of Animal Science, Michigan State University,
East Lansing, Michigan, USA

CHRISTINA S. PETERSSON-WOLFE, MSc, PhD
Associate Professor, Department of Dairy Science, Virginia Tech, Blacksburg, Virginia,
USA

AUTHORS

PAMELA R.F. ADKINS, DVM, PhD
Department of Veterinary Medicine and Surgery, University of Missouri, Columbia,
Missouri, USA

GEOFFREY E. DAHL, PhD
Harriet B. Weeks Professor, Department of Animal Sciences, Institute of Food and
Agricultural Sciences, University of Florida, Gainesville, Florida, USA

SANDRA M. GODDEN, DVM, DVSc
Professor, Department of Veterinary Population Medicine, College of Veterinary Medicine,
University of Minnesota, St Paul, Minnesota, USA

LAURA L. HERNANDEZ, PhD
Associate Professor, Department of Dairy Science, University of Wisconsin-Madison,
Madison, Wisconsin, USA

ALFONSO LAGO, DVM, PhD
Diplomate, American Board of Veterinary Practitioners (Dairy Practice); Chief Science
Officer, Research and Development Department, DairyExperts, Tulare, California, USA

KENNETH E. LESLIE, DVM, MSc
Professor Emeritus, Department of Population Medicine, University of Guelph, Guelph,
Ontario, Canada

STEPHANIE A. METZGER, PhD
Departments of Dairy Science, and Medical Microbiology and Immunology, University of
Wisconsin-Madison, Madison, Wisconsin, USA

JOHN R. MIDDLETON, DVM, PhD
Department of Veterinary Medicine and Surgery, University of Missouri, Columbia, Missouri, USA

JOHN F. PENRY, BVSc, MVS, PhD
Member, Australian and New Zealand College of Veterinary Scientists, Cattle Chapter; Cognosco-Anexa FVC, Morrinsville, New Zealand

CHRISTINA S. PETERSSON-WOLFE, MSc, PhD
Associate Professor, Department of Dairy Science, Virginia Tech, Blacksburg, Virginia, USA

PAMELA L. RUEGG, DVM, MPVM
Professor and Chairperson, Department of Animal Science, Michigan State University, East Lansing, Michigan, USA

GEORGE E. SHOOK, PhD
Department of Dairy Science, University of Wisconsin-Madison, Madison, Wisconsin, USA

LORRAINE M. SORDILLO, MS, PhD
College of Veterinary Medicine, Michigan State University, East Lansing, Michigan, USA

GARRET SUEN, PhD
Associate Professor, Department of Bacteriology, University of Wisconsin-Madison, Madison, Wisconsin, USA

TURNER H. SWARTZ, PhD
Postdoctoral Research Associate, Department of Dairy Science, Virginia Tech, Blacksburg, Virginia, USA

KENT A. WEIGEL, PhD
Department of Dairy Science, University of Wisconsin-Madison, Madison, Wisconsin, USA

JOHN R. WENZ, DVM, MS
Associate Professor, Field Disease Investigation Unit, Department of Clinical Sciences, College of Veterinary Medicine, Washington State University, Pullman, Washington, USA

Contents

> The selective treatment of clinical mastitis based on culture results can reduce antibiotic use by more than 50% without sacrificing treatment efficacy. Local laboratories reporting results in a 24-hour period, or adoption of on-farm milk culture systems, allow producers to make strategic treatment decisions. On-farm culture systems are most reliable when used to classify infections in broad diagnostic categories such as no growth, gram-positive, or gram-negative growth. Diagnostic accuracy is crucial for on-farm culture systems to be efficacious and economically advantageous. Quality assurance is necessary for the success of on-farm culture systems.

> Treatment of bovine mastitis is the most common reason that antibiotics are used for adult dairy cows. Although antibiotics are essential to treat severe cases of clinical mastitis, using antibiotics to treat many cases of non-severe clinical mastitis does not result in improved bacteriologic or clinical outcomes. Mastitis treatment protocols should be pathogen specific; no antimicrobial therapy is recommended for many culture-negative or gram-negative cases when detected. Before withholding antibiotic therapy, it is important to assess the ability of affected cows to mount a successful immune response. When the immune system is compromised, antimicrobial therapy may be recommended.

> The milk microbiota is an intriguing area of research because milk with no bacterial growth in culture was long thought to be sterile. Recent DNA sequencing techniques have been developed that do not require bacteria to be culturable, and DNA from new bacteria have been reported in milk from dairy cow mammary glands with or without mastitis. Methodologies and results vary among research groups, and not enough is known about the milk microbiota for the results to be used for diagnosis or prognosis of mastitis.

Automatic milking systems, or robotic milking systems, are now well established as a milk harvesting technology in Europe, North America and Australasia. This system is quarter based harvesting where human activity is not routinely required for milking or initial mastitis detection activities. Mastitis risk factors common with conventional milking are: environmental contamination, teat congestion and teat hyperkeratosis risk. The risk factors which differ include: pre-milking preparation, impact formation, and overmilking risk. Mastitis detection technology varies between automatic milking unit types, but all should be characterised by test sensitivity, false alert rate and the gold standard used for test assessment.

Mastitis is a prevalent and costly disease on dairy farms. Improved management and hygiene can reduce the risk of infection by contagious or environmental pathogens, and genetic selection can confer permanent improvement in mastitis resistance. National veterinary recording systems in the Nordic countries have allowed direct selection for sire families with low incidence of clinical mastitis for 3 decades, whereas other countries have practiced indirect selection for lower somatic cell count. Recently, pooling of producer-recorded data from on-farm herd management software programs has enabled selection for reduced incidence of clinical mastitis in the United States and other leading dairy countries.

Heat stress abatement is not difficult to implement, and at a minimum all cows should have shade access regardless of housing or pasture access. Active cooling of lactating cows and dry cows can have dramatic effects on productive function and enhance immune status as well. Whereas the method of abatement may vary depending on humidity conditions at a particular location, cooling can be achieved in any environment. Therefore, producers should emphasize appropriate heat stress abatement throughout the production cycle to improve productivity and health, including limiting mastitis.

A diagnosis of mastitis is based on clinical observations or direct/indirect measures of the inflammatory response to infection, whereas a diagnosis of an intramammary infection is based on identification of the infectious agent. Somatic cell count/somatic cell score are common diagnostic tests for the detection of subclinical mastitis. Culture and polymerase chain reaction can be useful in the diagnosis of an intramammary infection; however, both have their advantages and disadvantages. Diagnosing the bacterial agent causing the intramammary infection can help to determine treatment and prevention strategies on the farm, which in turn can help to reduce incidence and prevalence.

Deriving value from clinical mastitis records requires accurate and consistent records and tools for efficient summary and analysis. Variation in clinical mastitis case definition or detection intensity across dairies does not preclude consistent data recording. Dairy management software can improve consistency of clinical mastitis records by prompting users for quarter(s) affected, treatment, and severity. User-defined record systems must establish and follow protocols for clinical mastitis data recording. All records must have the same information in the same order and use the same abbreviations. Clinical mastitis episodes should be recorded at the quarter level. Cow-level recording compromises record consistency and accuracy of outcomes.

The ability of dairy cattle to prevent infectious pathogens from causing mastitis is related to the efficiency of the mammary immune system. The primary roles of the bovine immune system are to prevent bacterial invasion of the mammary gland, eliminate existing infections, and restore mammary tissues to normal function. Mammary gland immunity uses a multifaceted network of physical, cellular, and soluble factors to protect the cow from the diverse array of mastitis-causing pathogens. Strategies to optimize mammary gland defenses can be an effective way to prevent the establishment of new intramammary infections and limit the use of antimicrobials to treat mastitis.

Despite the widespread implementation of mastitis control programs, mastitis is the most common and one of the costliest diseases in the dairy industry, with broad-ranging impacts and consequences. Recent technological advances have allowed researchers to assess the effects of mastitis on animal behavior and welfare, and the efficacy of mastitis treatments. Several nonsteroidal anti-inflammatory drugs are available as supportive therapies for clinical mastitis. This article focuses on recent advances in the assessment, therapy, and effects of mastitis on cow behavior and welfare.

VETERINARY CLINICS OF NORTH AMERICA: FOOD ANIMAL PRACTICE

SERIES OF RELATED INTEREST

Veterinary Clinics of North America: Equine Practice

THE CLINICS ARE NOW AVAILABLE ONLINE!
Access your subscription at:
www.theclinics.com

Preface

Mastitis in Dairy Cows

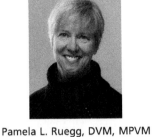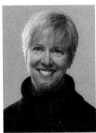

Pamela L. Ruegg, DVM, MPVM   Christina S. Petersson-Wolfe, MSc, PhD
Editors

Mastitis has always been an important disease of dairy cows, and its occurrence has a negative impact on animal well-being and farm profitability. Veterinarians have played an important role in controlling mastitis, but as the epidemiology of the disease has changed, our role has broadened. It is important to recognize that dramatic changes have occurred in farm technologies and herd structure, and public concerns about farm practices, such as antibiotic usage, have increased. All of these changes influence how veterinary practitioners interact with farmers to reduce the negative impact of mastitis on dairy farms.

For many decades, mastitis control was focused on reducing the prevalence of quarters infected with *Streptococcus agalactiae* and *Staphylococcus aureus*. The emphasis on controlling these pathogens was appropriate as a large proportion of cows were infected, and both product quality and profitability of farms were negatively impacted. To achieve this goal, researchers and veterinarians developed tests to detect subclinical mastitis, implemented the practice of comprehensive dry cow antibiotic therapy, identified preventive practices (such as the 5-point mastitis control plan) to limit spread of contagious pathogens among cows, and utilized intramammary antibiotic therapy to successfully treat quarters infected with *S agalactiae*. All of these control practices have formed the basis of how veterinarians are taught to effectively treat and prevent mastitis, and they have been successful. In the last decade, bulk tank somatic cell count values for US herds have consistently fallen, and the prevalence of subclinically infected quarters has been greatly reduced. On many modern farms, the challenges are different and are focused on control of a wider variety of opportunistic pathogens. In the United States, dramatic consolidation of dairy herds has occurred, and about 6% of herds are now producing about 60% of US milk. The remaining 94% of herds have had to be innovative to maintain a market for their milk and are under increasing pressure to adopt new technologies to become increasingly efficient.

Vet Clin Food Anim 34 (2018) ix–x
https://doi.org/10.1016/j.cvfa.2018.08.001
0749-0720/18/© 2018 Published by Elsevier Inc.   **vetfood.theclinics.com**

In this issue of *Veterinary Clinics of North America: Food Animal Practice*, we have invited authors to contribute articles that address many of these emerging concerns. Several articles focus on how veterinarians can use or understand new technologies, including new diagnostic methods and use of automatic milking systems. Other articles address the challenge of ensuring and documenting responsible antibiotic usage on dairy farms. The important issues of animal welfare and the role of heat stress and immunological responses to intramammary infection are also reviewed by leading researchers in these areas. We hope that the articles contributed by these outstanding authors will be of use to practicing veterinarians as they work with dairy farmers to meet today's challenges.

Pamela L. Ruegg, DVM, MPVM
Department of Animal Science
Michigan State University
474 South Shaw Lane
East Lansing, MI 48864, USA

Christina S. Petersson-Wolfe, MSc, PhD
Department of Dairy Science
Virginia Tech
175 West Campus Drive
Blacksburg, VA 24061, USA

E-mail addresses:
plruegg@msu.edu (P.L. Ruegg)
milk@vt.edu (C.S. Petersson-Wolfe)

Use of Rapid Culture Systems to Guide Clinical Mastitis Treatment Decisions

Alfonso Lago, DVM, PhD[a],*, Sandra M. Godden, DVM, DVSc[b]

KEYWORDS

- Selective treatment of mastitis • Judicious use of antibiotics
- Reduction of antibiotic use • On-farm culture • Rapid culture systems

KEY POINTS

- The selective treatment of clinical mastitis based on culture results can reduce antibiotic use by more than 50% without sacrificing treatment efficacy.
- Dairy herds could incur considerable savings on treatment-related costs (discarded milk, drugs, and labor), especially if extended treatment durations are implemented.
- Local professional laboratories reporting results in a 24-hour period, or adoption of on-farm milk culture systems, allow producers to make strategic treatment decisions.
- On-farm culture systems are most reliable when used to classify infections in broad diagnostic categories, such as no growth, gram-positive, or gram-negative growth.
- Diagnostic accuracy is crucial for on-farm culture systems to be efficacious and economically advantageous. Quality assurance is necessary for the success of on-farm culture systems.

INTRODUCTION

Clinical mastitis in dairy cattle has significant ramifications, including adverse effects on cow health and welfare, financial losses to dairy farmers, and public health concerns because of the extensive use of antibiotics for treatment. Therefore, there is a need to implement effective management strategies that also allow for judicious use of antibiotics. Not all clinical mastitis cases benefit from antibiotic therapy; some cases may benefit from different treatment strategies to optimize cure (eg, short vs. long duration), whereas chronic or otherwise nonresponsive cases may be best managed through

Disclosure Statement: Dr S.M. Godden is a Professor of Dairy Population Medicine employed at the University of Minnesota, which is the current distributor for one commercial on-farm culture system reviewed in this article (Minnesota Easy Culture System II). Dr A. Lago has nothing to disclose.

[a] Research and Development Department, DairyExperts, 1814 Rothschild Street, Tulare, CA 93274, USA; [b] Department of Veterinary Population Medicine, College of Veterinary Medicine, University of Minnesota, 225 VMC, 1365 Gortner Avenue, St Paul, MN 55108, USA
* Corresponding author.
E-mail address: alfonso.lago@dairyexperts.com

other means (eg, dry off the quarter, segregate or cull the cow). The type of agent causing mastitis may be a major determinant of the treatment or management strategy selected. Thus, knowledge of the cause of each case of clinical mastitis before making a treatment decision could assist in selecting cases that will be treated with antibiotics and to determine the appropriate duration of therapy. However, this will require rapid and accurate diagnosis of the cause of mastitis. This article discusses cause-based treatment decisions founded on the aim of improving antibiotic stewardship and selecting treatment strategies with a view to optimizing cure. The accuracy and efficacy of culture-based treatment decisions using rapid culture systems and guidelines for the implementation of on-farm culture systems are reviewed.

JUSTIFICATION
Treatment Efficacy for Nonsevere Cases of Clinical Mastitis Caused by Gram-Negative Bacteria

Gram-negative bacteria tend to have a more complex layering in their cell wall structure. Although the cell wall does contain peptidoglycans, it also contains a complex and species unique lipopolysaccharide (LPS) layer.[1] LPS, or endotoxin, typically elicits an acute immune response in an infected animal. *Escherichia coli* is perhaps the primary gram-negative contributor to mastitis in dairy cows. Because many antibiotics target peptidoglycans, treatment of gram-negative bacteria proves difficult in comparison to gram-positive pathogens.[2] The efficacy of antibiotics was also questioned on the basis of knowledge of the pathophysiology of coliform mastitis,[2,3] which includes the spontaneous rapid drop of milk bacterial counts 8 to 24 hours after infection and the risk of a massive release of bacterial endotoxins induced by antimicrobials.[2,4-6] Clinical recognition of coliform mastitis usually occurs after peak bacterial numbers have been attained.[3,6,7] Thus, by the time therapy is initiated, maximal release of endotoxin has likely already occurred. The additional release of endotoxins resulting from antibiotic therapy raises concerns regarding the advantages of antibacterial therapy in alleviating the effects of acute coliform mastitis. *Klebsiella* spp infections last significantly longer than *E coli* infections and are not likely to respond to antibiotic treatment.[8,9]

Most, but not all, field trials and trials with experimentally induced coliform mastitis have failed to prove the efficacy of antimicrobial treatment. In a retrospective cohort study, bacteriologic spontaneous cure rates for untreated cases of *E coli* and *Klebsiella* spp were high, 85%.[10] Cows experimentally challenged with *E coli* and treated with intramammary (IMM) gentamicin every 14 hours did not have lower peak bacterial concentrations in milk, duration of infection, convalescent somatic cell or serum albumin concentrations in milk, or rectal temperatures, as compared with the untreated challenged cows.[3] In a clinical trial conducted on 3 California dairies, bacteriologic cure and clinical cure did not differ after treatment with amoxicillin, cephapirin, or oxytocin (non-antibacterial) for nonsevere clinical mastitis cases caused by coliforms.[11] Another field trial intended to determine the efficacy of 4 methods (IMM amoxicillin, frequent milk-out, a combined IMM amoxicillin and frequent milk-out, and no treatment) for managing mild to moderate clinical mastitis in a university dairy herd. Treatment method appeared to have little effect on clinical and microbiological cures, milk production, disease progression, and California Mastitis Tests scores for *E coli* mastitis, because nearly all cases recovered within a short timeframe.[9] Similarly, one other field study found that IMM therapy using experimental antibiotic products was ineffective for gram-negative IMM infections.[12]

Some controversy over the use of antibiotic treatment of coliform mastitis was introduced by a controlled experiment at the University of Illinois dairy, showing that clinical and bacteriologic cure rates were significantly higher in clinical mastitis cases caused by environmental streptococci or coliform bacteria when treated by IMM administration of cephapirin and/or intravenous administration of oxytetracycline.[13] However, the interpretation of that study is problematic because data from 2 very different bacteriologic groups, streptococci and coliforms, had been pooled. A more recent study reported that nonsevere clinical gram-negative mastitis cases treated with ceftiofur hydrochloride had a significant increase in bacteriologic cure compared with nontreated controls in animals infected with *E coli* or *Klebsiella* spp.[14] In this study, in order to consider a bacteriologic cure, 2 posttreatment milk samples needed to be available for culture. When no or only one milk sample was present, cases were classified as a bacteriologic failure. These cases represented 11% of the cases in the treated group and 25% of the cases in the nontreated group. The result was that more mastitis cases were classified as bacteriologic failures in the nontreated group because posttreatment milk samples were not available for culture. Finally, when looking at economically based outcomes, this study reported no significant differences between treated and nontreated animals in future milk production or linear score after the clinical mastitis event (**Table 1**).

Efficacy of Extended Therapy for Clinical Mastitis Caused by Staphylococcus aureus and Environmental Streptococci

Knowing the cause of clinical mastitis not only allows for selective treatment decisions for clinical mastitis (ie, treat/no treat) but also may guide differential treatment decisions in terms of type of antibiotic selected or treatment duration. There is considerable evidence that longer treatment durations result in higher bacteriologic cures for pathogens that have the ability to invade secretory tissue (eg, *S aureus* and some environmental streptococcus). *S aureus* mastitis poses a therapeutic challenge because of several factors related to pathogenesis. Reported cure rates for *S aureus* mastitis vary considerably depending on certain cow, pathogen, and treatment-related factors.[15] Cure rates decrease with increasing age of the cow, increasing somatic cell count (SCC), increasing duration of infection, increasing bacterial colony counts in milk before treatment, and increasing number of quarters infected. Also the probability of cure is lower for β-lactamase–producing, penicillin-resistant *S aureus* than for penicillin-sensitive *S aureus*. Likewise, the probability of cure for *Streptococcus uberis* was higher among first- and second-parity animals than among older cows and was higher in animals with a single elevated cow-level SCC than in animals with multiple high SCC records.[16] One important factor affecting cure is treatment duration.

Table 1
Bacteriologic and clinical cure for coliform clinical mastitis either treated or not treated with intramammary antibiotics

Study	Sample Size	Antibiotic	Bacteriologic Cure (%)		Clinical Cure (%)	
			Treated	Nontreated	Treated	Nontreated
Guterbock et al,[11] 1993	94 cases in 3 herds	Amoxicillin Cephapirin	38 50	57 —	68 50	63 —
Morin et al,[13] 1998	172 cases in 1 herd	Cephapirin	87	72	47	15
Roberson et al,[9] 2004	38 cases in 1 herd	Amoxicillin	64	75	59	50
Schukken et al,[14] 2011	104 cases in 5 herds	Ceftiofur	76	38	54	46

Increased duration of treatment is associated with increased chance of cure.[15] Similarly, longer treatment durations have improved cure rates for *S uberis*. **Table 2** summarizes studies evaluating different treatment durations.

Shift in Cause of Clinical Mastitis Cases

In the last few decades in many herds, there has been a shift in the cause of clinical mastitis from Gram positives to Gram negatives and cases that yield no bacteria growth, cases for which there is a questionable need for antibiotic therapy. North American publications from the last decade have reported frequency distributions averaging 24% (range from 7% to 40%) for clinical cases for which coliforms were isolated and 35% (range from 21% to 56%) for clinical cases for which bacteria were not isolated (no bacterial growth) (**Table 3**). Other pathogens, such as yeast, *Pseudomonas*, *Mycoplasma*, *Nocardia*, and *Prototheca*, are not susceptible to antibiotics and are isolated in a smaller percentage of all clinical mastitis cases.

There may be multiple explanations for a "no-growth" result when culturing milk from clinical cases, including (a) mastitis was due to a noninfectious origin; (b) the quarter sampled was infected, but the cow's immune system had already eliminated the infection before the sample was taken (common in gram-negative infections)[3,6,7]; (c) microorganism presence was below detection thresholds[35]; (d) bacteria or other organism causing the mastitis does not grow in standard media culture or under the conditions offered (eg, viruses, anaerobic bacteria), or presence of substances in the milk decreasing the viability of bacteria in culture[36]; or (e) errors in sample collection, storage, culture media preservation, culture technique, incubation conditions, plate reading, and so forth.

Table 2
Bacteriologic cure for *Staphylococcus aureus* and *Streptococcus uberis* depending on the duration of the treatment

Study	Sample Size	Type	Antibiotic	Short Duration Days	Short Duration Cure (%)	Long Duration Days	Long Duration Cure (%)
Staphylococcus aureus							
Sol et al,[17] 2000	103 cases in 100 herds	Clinical	Various	2	48	4	74
Deluyker et al,[18] 2001	76 cases in 57 herds	Subclinical	Pirlimycin	2	25	8	51
		Subclinical	Pirlimycin	2	13	5	31
Ziv and Storper,[19] 1985		Subclinical	Penicillin	2	49	4	57
			Penethamate	2	63	4	69
			Methicillin	2	24	4	32
			Thamethicillin	2	20	4	49
Oliver et al,[20] 2004	38 cases in 3 herds	Subclinical	Ceftiofur	2	7	5	17
						8	36
Streptococcus uberis							
Oliver et al,[21] 2004	37 cases in 1 herd	Clinical	Ceftiofur	2	43	5	88
						8	100
Deluyker et al,[18] 2001	99 cases in 57 herds	Subclinical	Pirlimycin	2	24	8	75
Gillespie et al,[22] 2002	36 cases in 2 herds	Subclinical	Pirlimycin	2	50	5	83
						8	100
Oliver et al,[20] 2004	18 cases in 3 herds	Subclinical	Ceftiofur	2	17	5	56
						8	67

Table 3
Distribution of pathogens causing clinical mastitis from recent North American studies

Study	Sample Size	Strep ag or Staph aureus (%)	Non-aureus Staph (%)	Env Strep (%)	Coliform (%)	Other (%)	No Growth (%)
Vasquez et al,[23] 2017	489 cases in 1 herd	0	2	32	34	2	30
Vasquez et al,[24] 2016	596 cases in 6 herds	7	2	20	19	19	33
Lago et al,[25] 2016	223 cases in 1 herd	0	12	22	7	3	56
Tovar et al,[26] 2016	473 cases in 1 herd	0	19	30	10	4	37
Oliveira et al,[27] 2013	741 cases in 50 herds	3	6	13	37	14	27
Schukken et al,[28] 2013	296 cases in 7 herds	3	3	29	24	14	28
MacDonald,[29] 2011	675 cases in 48 herds	14	5	21	9	23	28
Lago et al,[30] 2011	449 cases in 8 herds	7	9	14	24	12	34
Pinzón-Sánchez and Ruegg,[31] 2011	143 cases in 4 herds	1	3	18	30	6	42
Bar et al,[32] 2007	2965 cases in 5 herds	5	3	21	40	10	21
Olde Riekerink et al,[33] 2008	2850 cases in 106 herds	11	6	16	14	7	46
Hoe and Ruegg,[34] 2005	217 cases in 4 herds	0	14	24	25	8	29

ON-FARM CULTURE SYSTEMS

As previously reported, more than half of mild and moderate clinical mastitis cases yield no bacterial growth or gram-negative bacteria and may not require antibiotic therapy. Conversely, IMM antibiotic therapy is routinely recommended for infections caused by gram-positive organisms, such as *Streptococcus agalactiae*, and environmental streptococci species. Management of *S aureus* cases may depend on the likelihood for cure: producers may opt to try IMM antibiotic therapy for newer cases but may decide to manage chronic cases differently using strategies such as segregation, drying off the quarter, or culling the cow. Consequently, to promote good antibiotic steward- ship and to optimize chances for a cure, clinical mastitis treatment decisions should be based on knowing the cause of infection. However, laboratory culture has not been routinely used by many dairies for this purpose primarily because of the time delay be- tween submission of milk samples and reporting of results. Providing faster laboratory results from local veterinary clinics or regional laboratories, or adoption of rapid on-farm milk culture (OFC) systems, could allow producers to make strategic treatment deci- sions for clinical mastitis cases, based on knowing the pathogen or pathogen group involved. Many different rapid culture systems are available worldwide. The following section discusses validation studies to describe the test characteristics and overall use- fulness of several commercially available OFC systems in North America.

Tests Characteristics of Rapid Culture Systems to Guide Clinical Mastitis Treatment Decisions

Minnesota easy culture system II
The Minnesota Easy Culture System II (University of Minnesota, St. Paul, MN, USA) is a commercial OFC system offering 2 different types of selective culture media systems. The Bi-plate system is a plate with 2 different types of agar: MacConkey agar on one- half selectively grows gram-negative organisms, whereas factor agar on the other half of the plate selectively grows gram-positive organisms (*Staphylococci* and *Strepto- cocci* or *Strep*-like species). Alternately, the Tri-plate system is a plate with 3 different types of agar: in addition to including MacConkey agar (gram-negative growth) and factor agar (gram-positive growth), it also includes a section of MTKT agar, which is selective for the growth of *Streptococci* or *Strep*-like species. Producers dip a sterile cotton swab into the milk sample and then apply it over the media surface (estimate 0.1 mL plating volume). The plate is incubated in an on-farm incubator at 37°C and is read at 18 to 24 hours. If no growth is observed, plates are rechecked after 48 hours and then discarded (**Figs. 1–3**).

The Bi-plate test characteristics have been evaluated in several different studies by comparing OFC system results against results from standard bacteriologic culture procedures.[37–40] Lago[38] evaluated the Bi-Plate in clinical mastitis samples in 8 different farms. If the operator's goal was to provide IMM antibiotic therapy to gram-positive infections but not to treat gram-negative or "no growth" cases, then the Bi-plate system would have resulted in the correct treatment decision 81% of the time. Specifically, the Bi-plate system had a sensitivity to identify gram-positive growth of 78% and a specificity of 83%. On-farm test characteristics from this study were comparable to 2 other reports in which the Bi-plate was evaluated to identify gram-positive growth in a laboratory setting by 2 readers.[37,40] However, higher sensi- tivity and lower specificity were reported in a different report.[39] The Bi-plate had a sensitivity of 98% and a specificity of 68%.

When the same samples evaluated by Hochhalter and colleagues[37] were plated on the Tri-plate on-farm culture system in a laboratory setting and read by 2 technicians,

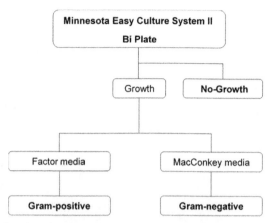

Fig. 1. Flowchart for identification of mastitis organisms using the Minnesota Easy Culture System II Bi-Plate. (*Adapted from* Minnesota Easy® Culture System II User's Manual. University of Minnesota, Saint Paul (MN); 2013, with permission.)

the sensitivity and specificity of the Tri-plate to detect gram-positive growth was 78%, as compared with results from traditional laboratory culture methods.[41] When evaluated for ability to differentiate Staphylococci from Streptococci growth, the Tri-plate had a sensitivity and specificity of 78% to 84% and 67% to 74%, respectively. In a different study validating the Tri-plate in a laboratory setting by a trained laboratory technician,[42] the test characteristics of the Tri-plate was reported when used to identify *S aureus*, and to differentiate streptococcal growth from other Gram-positive

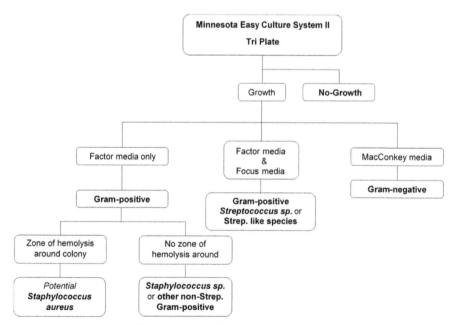

Fig. 2. Flowchart for identification of mastitis organisms using the Minnesota Easy Culture System II Tri-Plate. (*Adapted from* Minnesota Easy® Culture System II User's Manual. University of Minnesota, Saint Paul (MN); 2013, with permission.)

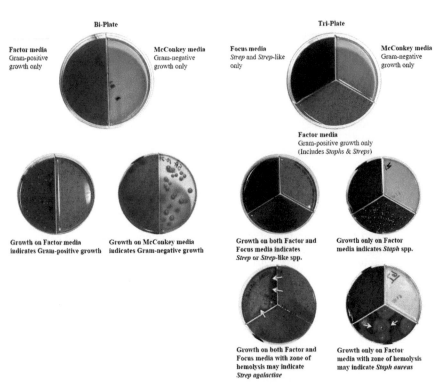

Fig. 3. Bi-Plate and Tri-Plate interpretation. (*Adapted from* Minnesota Easy® Culture System II User's Manual. University of Minnesota, Saint Paul (MN); 2013, with permission.)

growth in samples from clinical mastitis cases. For *S aureus*, the sensitivity was 98% and specificity was 82%. For differentiation of streptococcal growth, the sensitivity was 93% and the specificity was 90%.

Royster and colleagues[40] also evaluated both the Bi-plate and Tri-plate in a laboratory setting with 2 untrained student technicians interpreting the plates to identify the following diagnostic categories: no bacterial growth, Gram positive, Gram negative, Staphylococci, Streptococci, *S agalactiae*, *Streptococcus dysgalactiae*, *S uberis*, *Aerococcus* spp, *Enterococcus* spp, *S aureus*, coagulase-negative staphylococci, *E coli*, and *Klebsiella* spp. Although specificity and negative predictive values were generally high (>80%) for each diagnostic category, sensitivity and positive predictive values were intermediate (60%–80%) or high (>80%) for the broad categories of no growth, Gram positives and Gram negatives, Staphylococci growth, Streptococci growth, and *S aureus*, but were generally lower (<60%) for most other species specific. The aforementioned Bi-plate and Tri-plate validation studies reported interreader agreement from moderate to excellent for the general categories of growth, Gram positives, and Gram negatives.

In conclusion, Bi-plate and Tri-plate on-farm culture systems are most reliable when used to classify infections in broad diagnostic categories such as no growth, Gram positives, or gram-negative growth. Both Bi-plate and Tri-plate have moderate ability to identify and differentiate infections as being caused by Staphylococci and Streptococci. Finally, perhaps with the exception of *S aureus*, they should not be used to attempt to diagnose the cause of mastitis infections at the species level. Because of the moderate accuracy for diagnosis of *S aureus*, producers with a suspect *S aureus* result on the Bi-plate and Tri-plate are still encouraged to run a confirmatory test (eg, tube coagulase test) before making a case management decision (**Table 4**).[40]

3M Petrifilm system

The 3M Petrifilm Aerobic count plate and 3M Petrifilm Coliform count plate are ready-made selective culture media systems that are used for counting aerobic or coliform bacteria from food products.[43] They require a 24-hour incubation period and have an indicator dye that facilitates colony counting. When this culture system was evaluated to identify gram-positive bacteria in clinical mastitis samples at the laboratory, performed similarly to the Minnesota Easy Culture Bi-Plate System, a cut-point of greater than 5 colonies needed to be used to declare infection using the 3M Petrifilm Aerobic count plate and a cut-point of less than 20 colonies in the Coliform count plate needed to be used to declare a gram-positive infection.[39] The 3M Petrifilm test system had a sensitivity to identify gram-positive infections of 94% and a specificity of 70%. In addition to the need of establishing a cut-point for the 3M Petrifilm system to perform similarly to the Bi-plate on-farm culture system, investigators reported that because of artifact created by mastitis debris, samples were subsequently diluted 1:10 with sterile water before being placed on the 3M Petrifilm. This need for dilution might make adoption of the 3M Petrifilm system more difficult to implement on some farms (**Figs. 4** and **5**).

When the 3M Petrifilm system Aerobic and Coliform count plates were evaluated on-farm, they performed poorly.[29] Overall, sensitivity and specificity were 64% and 48%, respectively. However, the test performance varied widely among farms according to the frequency of use. A large proportion of herds enrolled in the clinical trial was small in size and used OFC less than once per month. Herds using OFC at least once per month reached a sensitivity and specificity of 82% and 46%, respectively. In general, some dairy producers reported that colony interpretation was a challenge. Investigators reported that actual growth may take on a wide range of patterns from small numbers of clearly visible, dark red colonies to diffuse, light-colored colonies instead of clearly demarcated colonies. Clots in milk applied to Coliform count 3M Petrifilm may also turn pink in color and could be mistaken for colony growth. Application of too much pressure on the spreaders used to spread the milk sample evenly across

Table 4
Sensitivity, specificity, positive predictive values, and negative predictive values of the Minnesota Easy Culture Bi-Plate System Bi-Plate and Tri-Plate in order to identify gram-positive bacterial growth in quarter secretion samples from clinical mastitis cases during lactation

Study	Culture System	Test Validation Location	Test Characteristics (%) Se	Sp	Predictive Values (%) PPV	NPV
Lago,[38] 2011	Bi-Plate	On farm	78	83	74	86
Royster et al,[40] 2014	Bi-Plate	In laboratory (Reader 1)	85	79	92	64
		In laboratory (Reader 2)	80	87	95	58
Royster et al,[40] 2014	Tri-Plate	In laboratory (Reader 1)	86	76	91	66
		In laboratory (Reader 2)	80	93	97	62
McCarron et al,[39] 2009	Bi-Plate	In laboratory	98	68	78	96
McCarron et al,[39] 2009	Bi-Plate	In laboratory	77	78	68	85
Jones et al,[41] 2006	Tri-Plate	In laboratory	78	78	71	84

Abbreviations: NPV, negative predictive values; PPV, positive predictive values; Se, sensitivity; Sp, specificity.

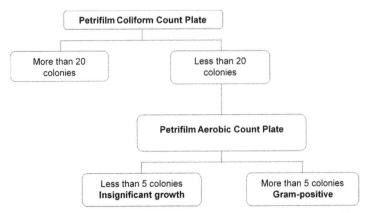

```
┌─────────────────────────────────────┐
│    Petrifilm Coliform Count Plate    │
└─────────────────────────────────────┘
```

```
┌──────────────────┐        ┌──────────────────┐
│   More than 20   │        │   Less than 20   │
│     colonies     │        │     colonies     │
└──────────────────┘        └──────────────────┘
```

```
┌─────────────────────────────────────┐
│    Petrifilm Aerobic Count Plate     │
└─────────────────────────────────────┘
```

```
┌─────────────────────────┐   ┌─────────────────────────┐
│   Less than 5 colonies  │   │   More than 5 colonies  │
│   Insignificant growth  │   │      Gram-positive      │
└─────────────────────────┘   └─────────────────────────┘
```

Fig. 4. Flowchart for identification of mastitis organisms using the 3M Petrifilm On-Farm Culture System. (*Data from* McCarron JL, Keefe GP, McKenna SL, et al. Evaluation of the University of Minnesota Tri-plate and 3M Petrifilm for the isolation of *Staphylococcus aureus* and *Streptococcus* species from clinically mastitic milk samples. J Dairy Sci 2009;92:5326–33.)

the 3M Petrifilm plate caused concentration of the milk sample around the outer ring of the culture surface with growth appearing as a pink ring rather than individual colonies, which were mistaken as absence of growth by some dairy producers. The investigators concluded that training and provision of comprehensive interpretation guides showing a variety of possible growth patterns on 3M Petrifilm could improve the accuracy of the on-farm culture system in the future. An additional evaluation of the 3M Petrifilm system was also conducted on a German dairy farm, but both preparation and evaluation of the 3M Petrifilm plates were conducted by a trained researcher at the farm.[44] The sensitivity and specificity of the 3M Petrifilm to identify gram-positive growth was 85% and 75%, respectively. The investigators concluded that results indicate that the 3M Petrifilm system is suitable for therapeutic decision making at the farm level or in veterinary practice.

The 3M Petrifilm Staph Express Count Plate (STX) is designed to be selective and differential for *Staphylococcus* spp. The 3M Petrifilm produces results within 24 ± 2 hours of incubation. Red-violet colonies on the plate are *S aureus*.[43] A sensitivity of 88% and specificity of 66% were reported for isolation of *S aureus* when evaluated in a laboratory setting.[44] A similar sensitivity (95%) and specificity (76%) were reported when evaluated in similar conditions.[42] However, the diagnosis of *S aureus* using the 3M Petrifilm STX method is highly dependent on the ability of the individual reading

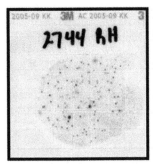
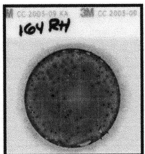
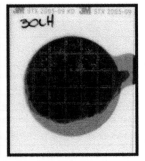

Fig. 5. 3M Petrifilm System Plates. (Used with permission from 3M, St Paul, MN.)

the test to observe variations in colony color.[45] In cases where the color of the colonies is not easily identified or when colonies other than red-violet are present on the plate, the 3M Petrifilm STX disk, which requires 3 hours of additional incubation, may be used to identify *S aureus*. Thus, it was reported an improvement in specificity from 76% to 93% and similar sensitivity (95% vs 92%) when using the STX disk **(Table 5)**.[42]

Other rapid culture systems

Chromogenic media have also been used for identification of microorganisms from mastitic milk samples. As an example, the Accumast system uses 3 selective chromogenic media to identify specific bacteria or group of bacteria (FERA Animal Health LCC, Ithaca, NY, USA). This system claims to be able identify *S aureus*, *Staphylococcus* spp, *Streptococcus* spp, *Enterococcus* spp or *Lactococcus* spp, *Klebsiella* spp, *Enterobacter* spp or *Serratia* spp, *E coli*, other gram-negative bacteria, and milk samples with no bacterial growth. Two validation studies have thus far investigated the diagnostic utility of this system for the detection of several pathogen groups and some, but not all, of the bacterial species listed above.[46,47] For example, one study of 538 milk samples collected from cows with clinical mastitis reported the test characteristics of the Accumast system to identify growth versus no growth; gram-negative growth; gram-positive growth; *E coli*, Pseudomonas sp, other Gram-negatives, *Enterococcus* spp, *Staphylococcus* spp, *S aureus*, and *Streptococcus* spp.[46] In this study, the overall sensitivity and specificity of the system to identify bacterial growth were reported to be 82.3% and 89.9%, respectively. Further independent validation of the Accumast system is needed for several pathogens, and particularly for *S aureus*, because the studies that have been published included only 7 and 2 milk samples, respectively, that were positive for this pathogen **(Figs. 6 and 7)**.[46,47]

CHROMagar Mastitis (CHROMagar, Paris, France) is another chromogenic medium and was also compared in a laboratory setting to 3 other on-farm culture media (Minnesota Easy Culture System Tri-plate; VétoRapid, Vetoquinol, Hertogenbosch, The Netherlands; Hardy Tri-plate, Hardy Diagnostics, Santa Maria, CA, USA). All systems had a similar sensitivity and specificity to detect gram-positive and gram-negative growth, as well as no-growth.[48]

Dry Culture Media (NeoFilm; Neogen Corporation, MI, USA) quantify and identify bacterial class (Gram positive or Gram negative)" with "NeoFilm® Dry Culture Media (Neogen Corporation, Lansing, MI, USA) quantify and identify bacterial class (Gram positive or Gram negative). When evaluated, on-farm agreed more than 82% of the time with laboratory results when determining if a milk sample was negative or yielded gram-negative or gram-positive bacteria.[49]

Table 5
Sensitivity, specificity, positive predictive values, and negative predictive values of the 3M Petrifilm System in order to identify gram-positive bacterial growth in quarter secretion samples from clinical mastitis cases during lactation

Study	Culture System	Test Validation Location	Test Characteristics (%)		Predictive Values (%)	
			Se	Sp	PPV	NPV
MacDonald,[29] 2011	3M Petrifilm	On farm	64	48	55	58
Mansion-de Vries et al,[44] 2014	3M Petrifilm	On farm[a]	85	75	70	88
McCarron et al,[39] 2009	3M Petrifilm	In laboratory	94	70	80	90

[a] The preparation and evaluation of the 3M Petrifilm plates was conducted by a trained researcher at the farm.

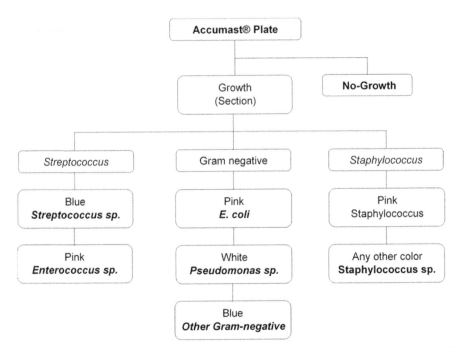

Fig. 6. Flowchart for identification of mastitis organisms using Accumast System. (*Adapted from* Ganda EK, Bisinotto RS, Decter DH, et al. Evaluation of an on-farm culture system (Accumast) for fast identification of milk pathogens associated with clinical mastitis in dairy cows. PLoS One 2016;11:e0155314; with permission.)

When choosing among rapid culture systems for potential adoption on farms or in local veterinary clinics, producers or veterinarians will need to consider such attributes as accuracy, cost, shelf life, necessary storage conditions, ease of use, and customer support provided by the manufacturer. However, most importantly, consideration must be given to what information is required of the test. For example, if the mastitis treatment protocol on a farm dictates that only gram-positive cases will be treated with antibiotic, then any rapid culture system that can differentiate between gram-positive growth (vs gram-negative or no growth) will be sufficient. Conversely, if treatment protocols require that more detailed information regarding the presence or absence of any particular pathogen group or bacterial species, in order to guide different treatment decisions, then a rapid culture system should be selected that allows for an accurate diagnosis to that desired level. Currently, no rapid culture system will allow for the diagnosis of some mastitis organisms that require special culture conditions or more advanced tests in order to identify the genus and species (eg, *Mycoplasma* spp).

Efficacy to Guide Clinical Mastitis Treatment Decisions

The previous discussion suggests that the selective treatment of clinical mastitis may represent a tremendous opportunity to reduce antibiotic use on commercial dairy farms without sacrificing the efficacy of treatment or the long-term health and production potential of the cow. Potential benefits of improved antibiotic stewardship could include reduced economic cost of therapy, reduced risk of antibiotic residues in milk, and a reduction in the potential risk for development of antibiotic resistance in mastitis pathogens. However, many of these potential benefits needed further evaluation to

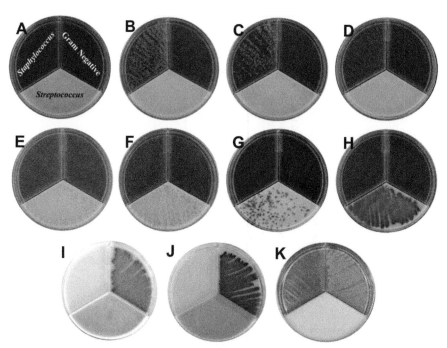

Fig. 7. Visual assessment of gram-positive and gram-negative bacterial growth on Accumast plates performed in laboratory. Pictures were taken on a dark background. Plate without bacteria (*A*), *S aureus* (*B*), *Staphylococcus epidermidis* (*C*), *Staphylococcus chromogenes* (*D*), *S agalactiae* (*E*), *Streptococcus dysgalactiae* (*F*), *S uberis* (*G*), *Enterococcus faecalis* (*H*), *E coli* (*I*),[a] *Klebsiella oxytoca* (*J*),[a] and *Pseudomonas aeruginosa* (*K*). [a] Pictures were taken on a light background. (*From* Ganda EK, Bisinotto RS, Decter DH, et al. Evaluation of an on-farm culture system (Accumast) for fast identification of milk pathogens associated with clinical mastitis in dairy cows. PLoS One 2016;11:e0155314; with permission.)

confirm and quantify the nature of these proposed benefits. The success of implementing an OFC system on a commercial dairy will depend not only on the accuracy of the OFC system being used but also on the strategic treatment decisions made based on OFC (eg, no IMM treatment of no growth or gram-negative cases) as well as whether there is a deleterious effect of a 1-day delay while waiting for OFC results before initiating IMM therapy in those quarters selected for antibiotic treatment. Outcomes from several clinical trials evaluating the effectiveness of selective treatment of clinical mastitis when compared with blanket therapy are reported in **Table 6.**

To assess the overall usefulness of adopting an OFC system, Lago and colleagues[30,50] conducted a multistate, multiherd clinical trial to evaluate the efficacy of using an OFC system to guide strategic treatment decisions in cows with clinical mastitis. The study was conducted in 8 commercial dairy farms ranging in size from 144 to 1795 cows from Minnesota, Wisconsin, and Ontario, Canada. A total of 422 cows affected with mild or moderate clinical mastitis in 449 quarters were randomly assigned to either (1) a positive-control treatment program or (2) an on-farm, culture-based treatment program (**Fig. 8**). Quarter cases assigned to the positive-control group received immediate on-label IMM treatment with cephapirin sodium (2 tubes, 12 hours apart). Quarters assigned to the culture-based treatment program were cultured on-farm using the Minnesota Easy Culture System II Bi-Plate and treated with IMM cephapirin sodium (2 tubes, 12 hours apart) after 18 to 24 hours

Table 6
Outcomes from several clinical trials evaluating the effectiveness of selective treatment of clinical mastitis when compared with blanket therapy

Study	Cases	Cases Treated (%)		Days to Clinical Cure (d)		Days out of Tank (d)		Bacteriologic Cure (%)		Recurrence (%)		Milk Yield (kg)		SCC Linear Score (cells/mL)		Culling/ Death (%)	
		B[a]	S[b]	B	S	B	S	B	S	B	S	B	S	B	S	B	S
Vasquez et al,[23] 2017	489 cases in 1 herd	100	32	4.8	4.5	8.8	5.8	—	—	—	—	35	35	4.2	4.3	12	10
Lago et al,[25] 2016	276 cases in 1 herd	100	28	3.1	3.5	6.7	5.7	77	77	25	13	—	—	—	—	14	7
Tovar et al,[26] 2016	475 cases in 1 herd	100	46	3.6	4.0	6.7	7.1	66	69	23	20	—	—	—	—	15	15
MacDonald,[29] 2011	747 cases in 48 herd	100	60	3.0	3.0	—	—	77[c]	75[c]	6.7	4.2	—	—	—	—	—	—
Lago et al,[30] 2011; Lago et al,[50] 2011	449 cases in 8 herds	100	44	2.7	3.2	5.9	5.2	71	60	35	43	30	31	4.2	4.4	28	32

[a] Blanket therapy.
[b] Selective treatment.
[c] Bacteriologic cure probability was calculated from the data reported in the article.

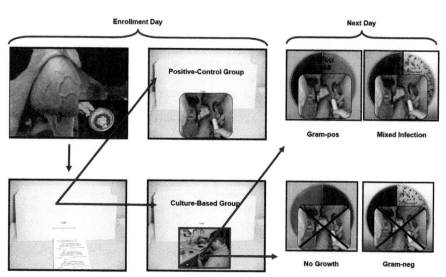

Fig. 8. Cows with mild and moderate clinical cases of mastitis were randomly assigned by opening a treatment assignment envelope to either the positive-control group or to the culture-based treatment group. Cases assigned to the positive-control group were treated with 2 tubes of cephapirin sodium 12 hours apart immediately after the milk sample was collected. Quarter cases assigned to the culture-based treatment group were cultured on the farm and treated the next day only if on-farm culture showed gram-positive or mixed growth. Quarters where bacteria were not isolated or with only gram-negative growth were not treated. (*Data from* Lago A, Godden SM, Bey R, et al. The selective treatment of clinical mastitis based on on-farm culture results: I. Effects on antibiotic use, milk withholding time, and short-term clinical and bacteriological outcomes. J Dairy Sci 2011;94(9):4441–56.)

of incubation if they showed gram-positive growth or a mixed infection. Quarters with gram-negative or no growth did not receive IMM therapy. The proportion of quarter cases assigned to positive-control and culture-based treatments that received IMM antibiotic therapy because of study assignment was 100% and 44%, respectively; the proportion of cases that received secondary antibiotic therapy was 36% and 19%, respectively, and the proportion of cases that received IMM antibiotic therapy because of either study assignment or secondary therapy was 100% and 51%, respectively.[30] A tendency existed for a decrease in the number of days in which milk was discarded from cows assigned to the culture-based treatment program versus cows assigned to the positive-control group (5.9 vs 5.2 days). No statistically significant differences existed between cases assigned to the positive-control and cases assigned to the culture-based treatment program in days to clinical cure (2.7 vs 3.2 days), bacteriologic cure risk within 21 days of enrollment (71% vs 60%), new IMM infection risk within 21 days of enrollment (50% vs 50%), and treatment failure risk (presence of infection, secondary treatment, clinical mastitis recurrence, or removal from herd within 21 days after enrollment; 81% vs 78%). When evaluating long-term outcomes of the aforementioned study, no differences existed between cases assigned to the positive-control program and cases assigned to the culture-based treatment program in risk and days for recurrence of clinical mastitis in the same quarter (35% and 78 days vs 43% and 82 days), linear somatic cell count (4.2 vs 4.4), daily milk production (30.0 vs 30.7 kg), and risk and days for culling or death events (28% and 160 days vs 32% and 137 days) for the rest of the lactation after enrollment of the clinical mastitis case.[50] In summary, the selective treatment of clinical mastitis based on on-farm culture resulted in no differences in long-term outcomes, such as recurrence of clinical mastitis in the same quarter, somatic cell count, milk production, and cow survival for the rest of the lactation after clinical mastitis. The investigators concluded that the use of an OFC system to guide the strategic treatment of clinical mastitis reduced IMM antibiotic use by half and tended to decrease milk withholding time by 1 day, without affecting short- or long-term health or performance of the quarter or cow.

MacDonald[29] also evaluated the selective treatment of gram-positive clinical mastitis using the 3M Petrifilm system for OFC. Again, primary antibiotic use was reduced by 40% in the culture-based treatment group with no difference in risk of receiving secondary antibiotic treatment compared with the control group. No significant differences were observed between groups for bacteriologic cure probability, risk of recurrence of infection, risk of developing a new infection, culling, or drying off. Even the average number of days to clinical cure was not different between groups; a significant difference was observed in the odds of clinical cure being lower for cases assigned to OFC. The difference was attributable to false negative diagnosis that resulted in a failure to treat cases caused by gram-positive pathogens. These results highlight the critical importance of the accuracy of on-farm culture in differentiating between Gram positive, Gram –negative, and no-growth for the selective treatment of clinical mastitis to be as efficacious as blanket therapy.

A potential limitation of the previous studies was that the label of the IMM antibiotic administered did not include efficacy claims against gram-negative bacteria. IMM antibiotic preparations, one containing ceftiofur and the other containing hetacillin potassium, are currently approved in the United States with a label that claims efficacy against clinical mastitis in lactating dairy cattle associated with *E coli*. Tovar and colleagues[26] assigned 425 cows with 475 mild or moderate clinical mastitis to either (a) a positive-control treatment group or (b) a laboratory culture–based treatment group. Quarter cases assigned to positive-control received blanket immediate IMM treatment with ceftiofur and was repeated once a day for a total of 3 days. Quarters assigned to culture-based treatment underwent culture over a 24-hour period at DairyExperts Laboratory (DairyExperts Inc, Tulare, CA, USA). Only quarters showing gram-positive growth were treated the next day with the same therapy as cases assigned to positive control. The selective treatment of only clinical mastitis cases from which gram-positive bacteria resulted in about half reduction both in the number of cases treated and in the number of IMM tubes used, but there was no reduction on days out of the tank. Furthermore, the withholding of antibiotic treatment did not have any deleterious effect on time for milk to return visibly normal, bacteriologic cure, new infection risk, clinical mastitis recurrence, or removal from the herd. Vasquez and colleagues[23] assigned 489 mild and moderate cases of clinical mastitis to the following 2 treatment groups: (a) blanket immediate IMM treatment with ceftiofur and repeated once a day for a total of 5 days or (b) laboratory culture–based treatment where only quarters from which *Staphylococcus* spp, *Streptococcus* spp, or *Enterococcus* spp were isolated received the following day 2 doses 12 hours apart of IMM treatment with cephapirin sodium. Only one-third of the cases of the pathogen-based treatment group received IMM antibiotics, resulting in a reduction of 3 days in the hospital. No significant differences existed between blanket therapy and pathogen-based therapy in days to clinical cure, milk production, test-day linear scores, or odds of survival 30 days after enrollment.

Lago and colleagues[25] conducted a study following the same study design as Tovar and colleagues[26] with the exception that in the laboratory culture–based treatment group only quarters showing environmental streptococci growth were treated. The selective treatment of only clinical mastitis cases from which environmental streptococci were isolated resulted in about a two-thirds reduction both in the number of cases treated and in the number of IMM tubes used, as well as a reduction of 1 day out of the tank. Furthermore, the withholding of antibiotic treatment did not increase the time for milk to return visibly normal or affect bacteriologic cure or new infection risk. Interestingly, clinical mastitis recurrence was significantly lower, and removal from herd tended to be lower when only environmental streptococci were treated with IMM antibiotics. To the authors' knowledge, this was the first study reporting health benefits from not treating all cases of clinical mastitis with antibiotics, and probably to any other disease in animals. Although this hypothesis requires further investigation, if findings from this study are found to be repeatable in future clinical trials, then selective treatment decisions and judicious use of antibiotics would be justifiable not just from the economics and public health concerns dimensions but also from an animal welfare one.

Other Applications of Rapid Culture Systems When Treating Clinical Mastitis

Differential mastitis treatment decisions

Differential treatment refers to following different antibiotic treatment strategies to optimize cure depending on the cause of infection (eg, selecting type of antibiotic, short vs. long duration). The economics of extended treatment therapy for S aureus or certain environmental streptococcus clinical mastitis (eg, S uberis) has been evaluated recently.[51–54] The profitability of extended duration was dependent on whether the bioeconomic model included the effect of pathogen transmission to uninfected cows, from cows that remained subclinically infected after treatment of clinical mastitis. Steeneveld and colleagues[51] evaluated the cost benefit of 3- and 5-day antibiotic treatment durations. Total costs included treatment costs (costs of antibiotics, milk withdrawal, and labor for the initial and recurrent cases of mastitis), milk production losses, and cost of culling, but not included was the probability of transmission to uninfected cows. Overall, the 3-day treatment had the lowest total costs. The benefits of lower costs for milk production losses and culling due to higher bacteriologic cure rates with the 5-day treatment did not outweigh the higher treatment costs. However, the cost differential for contagious pathogens to reach higher probability of cure was very small. For instance, treating S aureus clinical mastitis cases 5 days instead of 3 days increased the probability of cure by 25% and resulted only in an additional $5 cost even when the additional risk transmission was not considered in the model. When the impact of within-herd transmission of cows that remained subclinically infected was accounted for in this bioeconomic model, the risk of transmission was found to have the strongest association with the cost of clinical mastitis by contagious pathogens.[53] Halasa[53] concluded that low transmission rates of this pathogen for short-duration treatment (3 days) are the most cost-effective. However, in case of high transmission of contagious pathogens, longer duration treatments (5 days) are the most profitable.

Simultaneous treatment of quarters with subclinical mastitis

The economic value of lactation therapy for subclinical mastitis is generally considered to be limited because of the cost of milk discarded during the withdrawal period. However, the concurrent treatment of quarters affected with subclinical mastitis when treating other quarters already affected with clinical mastitis does not result in additional discarded milk. A high proportion of infected nonclinical quarters in cows with clinical mastitis would warrant the development of tools for the identification and treatment of those quarters. Lago and Silva-del-Rio[55] found that of all cows with clinical mastitis, 67% had bacteria isolated from at least one of the other 3 nonclinical quarters. If also considering the quarter affected with clinical mastitis, 82% of the cows had at least one-quarter infected (clinical or subclinical). Unfortunately, the CMT was not a sensitive enough tool for the identification of those subclinically infected quarters in cows with clinical mastitis. Thus, culture could be used to identify those other quarters subclinically infected.

Use of culture for secondary/extended treatment decisions

The duration of antibiotic therapy during a clinical case of mastitis depends on treatment protocols and/or on caregiver assessments. The identification of quarters still infected after the initial course of antibiotic treatment has been completed would allow for better characterization of cows that may benefit from extended or secondary therapy. Theoretically, culture could be used to identify quarters still infected after treatment. However, false negatives due to inhibition of bacterial growth because of antibiotic residues or false positives due to the presence of bacteria in death phase are expected. Lago and colleagues[56] evaluated the validity of the use of culture to evaluate bacteriologic cure the days after antibiotic IMM treatment. Culturing milk samples at days 1, 2, or 3 after treatment detected 67%, 60%, and 50% of the quarters that were still infected at days 7 or 14 after treatment (sensitivity) and classified as uninfected 79%, 93%, and 100% of the cases from which bacteria were not present at both 7 and 14 days (specificity). In summary, culturing milk 1 day after the last antibiotic treatment failed to identify one-third of persistent infections, probably due to the inhibitory effects of antibiotics (false negatives). However, false positives (isolation of bacteria days after treatment when bacteriologic cure still is going to happen) were not frequent.

MANAGING AN ON-FARM CULTURE LABORATORY

There are several considerations that go into setting up and operating a successful on-farm culture laboratory. For those farms that wish to set up their own OFC laboratory, recommendations for developing a successful system are provided below.

Location

The OFC laboratory should be located in a temperature-controlled room isolated from traffic and drafts solely dedicated to laboratory activities. It should have the following:

Workbench

Surfaces need to be easily cleaned and disinfected.

Incubator

Mastitis bacteria grow best at body temperature; therefore, the incubator must maintain its temperature at 37°C (98.6°F). The incubator should have an easy-to-read thermometer that allows monitoring that the incubator is operating properly. Mastitis bacteria grow best when the relative humidity is about 75%. This humidity is easily achieved by having a tray filled with water in the bottom of the incubator. Be sure to add water often. Finally, never turn off the incubator even if not used on a daily basis.

Refrigerators

It is preferable to have 2 refrigerators: a clean refrigerator to store media plates, or other supplies that need to be refrigerated, and a nonclean refrigerator to store milk samples and others.

Supplies

Supplies include disposable gloves, milk sample vials, racks for sample vials, sterile disposable cotton-tipped swabs, surface disinfectant, paper towels, and a waste container.

Record Keeping

There should be a log book to record sample date, cow ID, affected quarter, plating time, initial of technician plating, culture results, reading time, and initials of technician reading plates. Also, the refrigerators' temperature, incubator temperature, and presence or absence of water in the tray should be recorded on a daily basis.

Employee Training

Farm employees or veterinary technicians in charge of performing on-farm culture need to be properly trained and monitored. The training has to include a general introduction to microbiology and mastitis, equipment functioning and maintenance, new and used plates storage and discarding, milk sample collection and storage, plating procedures, incubation, reading of plates and interpreting results, and record keeping. The Minnesota Easy Culture System User's Guide[57] provides detailed information about laboratory setup, sample collection and handling, culturing procedures, and interpretation of culture results (https://www.vdl.umn.edu/services-fees/udder-health-mastitis/farm-culture).

Quality Assurance Needed for On-Farm Culture Systems

Ongoing quality assurance is a crucial part for the success of on-farm culture systems. As previously reviewed, accuracy of OFC results are critical for the economic viability of the system. Veterinarians or other qualified professionals should visit the dairy regularly (ie, weekly or biweekly basis) and review the following:

1. Milk sample collection and storage (ie, aseptic technique, rapid plating, or refrigeration)
2. Storage of new plates (ie, refrigerator temperature, plate stacks placed upside down)
3. Labeling of culture plates (ie, cow ID, quarters, and date)
4. Incubator functioning:
   a. Thermometer reading of 37°C (98.6°F)
   b. Presence of water in a tray located in the bottom of the incubator that aims to maintain relative humidity at about 75%
5. Plating technique (ie, no milk chunks, well-delimited swabbing between samples)
6. Placing of plates in the incubator (ie, upside down, not stacking more than 2 plates)
7. Time plates spent at the incubator (ie, minimum of 18 hours before first reading)
8. Reading of plates from that day with on-farm culture technician
9. Used plates should be stored in a refrigerator (different from the one where storing new plates) to
   a. Evaluate agreement with the on-farm culture technician results
   b. Additional testing (eg, colonies suspicious of being *S aureus*, *S agalactiae*, *Klebsiella* sp, *Prototheca* sp)
   c. Evaluate plating technique
   d. Identify contaminated samples
10. Calculate the frequency of contaminated cultures (objective would be <5%).

11. Observe hygiene practices (eg, no food or drinks at the laboratory or refrigerator, workers wear clean clothes and disposable gloves, laboratory benches are cleaned and disinfected)
12. Records evaluation
    a. Accurate entering of culture results
    b. Matching between culture results and treatment decisions
13. Discarding of plates (ie, autoclaving or contracting disposal services)
14. Farm staff working with OFC systems should periodically send milk samples to a local diagnostic laboratory for culture and then compare culture results with those obtained on farm.

Rapid Culture Services at Local Veterinary Clinics or Diagnostic Laboratories

If a designated clean laboratory space, proper training, ongoing quality assurance and retraining, and a committed, experienced, and properly trained individual are not in place, then the farm may not get good-quality information from the system (**Fig. 9**). Similarly, if farms have infrequent clinical mastitis cases, then the on-farm technician may not get enough experience to become comfortable or accurate when setting up cultures or interpreting the results when reading plates. In these situations, a perfect alternative to OFC is the use of professional laboratories or local veterinary clinics that can offer culture results within 24 hours to make treatment decisions at the farm.

SUMMARY

Cause-based treatment decisions for the selective treatment of clinical mastitis represent a tremendous opportunity to reduce antibiotic use on commercial dairy farms by more than 50% for the treatment of mild and moderate clinical mastitis cases without sacrificing the efficacy of treatment or the long-term health and production potential of the cow. Consequently, dairy herds could incur considerable savings on treatment-related costs (discarded milk, drugs, and labor), especially if extended treatment durations are

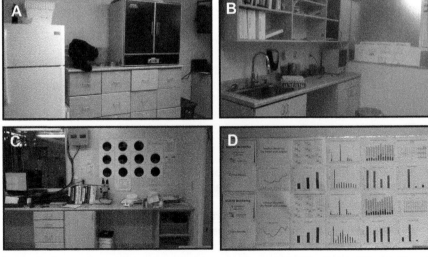

Fig. 9. On-farm culture laboratory. A refrigerator/freezer and incubator (A); workbench, sink, and bookshelves (B); computer for data entry and wall pictures providing guidance for plate reading (C); and mastitis epidemiology and laboratory monitoring graphs (D).

implemented. Additional benefits could include reduced risk of antibiotic residues in milk, and a reduction in the potential risk for development of antibiotic resistance in mastitis pathogens. Furthermore, differential treatment (adequate antibiotic selection or treatment duration depending on cause) could improve treatment efficacy.

Local professional laboratories can offer culture services, reporting results for treatment decisions in a 24-hour period, or adoption of OFC systems in select medium- to large-size dairies allows producers to make strategic treatment decisions for clinical mastitis cases, based on knowing the type of pathogen involved. On-farm culture systems are most reliable when used to classify infections in broad diagnostic categories, such as no growth, Gram positives, or gram-negative growth, but should not be used to diagnose the cause of mastitis infections at the species level. Diagnostic accuracy is crucial for on-farm culture systems to be efficacious and economically advantageous. Quality assurance with regular monitoring by a veterinarian or other qualified professional is necessary for the success of on-farm culture systems.

REFERENCES

1. Beveridge TJ. Structures of gram-negative cell walls and their derived membrane vesicles. J Bacteriol 1999;181:4725–33.
2. Pyörälä S, Kaartinen L, Kack H, et al. Efficacy of two therapy regimens for treatment of experimentally induced *Escherichia coli* mastitis in cows. J Dairy Sci 1994;77:453–61.
3. Erskine RJ, Wilson RC, Riddell MG Jr, et al. Intramammary gentamicin as a treatment for experimental *Escherichia coli* mastitis in cows. Am J Vet Res 1992;53:375–81.
4. Shenep JL, Mogan KA. Kinetics of endotoxin release during antibiotic therapy for experimental Gram-negative bacterial sepsis. J Infect Dis 1984;150:380–8.
5. Shenep JL, Barton RP, Mogan KA. Role of antibiotic class in the rate of liberation of endotoxin during therapy for experimental Gram-negative bacterial sepsis. J Infect Dis 1985;151:1012–8.
6. Hill AW, Shears AL, Hibbit KG. The pathogenesis of experimental *Escherichia coli* mastitis in newly calved dairy cows. Res Vet Sci 1979;26:97–101.
7. Anderson KL, Kindahl H, Petroni A, et al. Arachidonic acid metabolites in milk of cows during acute coliform mastitis. Am J Vet Res 1985;46:1573–7.
8. Smith KL, Todhunter DA, Schoenberger PS. Environmental mastitis: cause, prevalence, prevention. J Dairy Sci 1985;68:1531–53.
9. Roberson JR, Warnick LD, Moore G. Mild to moderate clinical mastitis: Efficacy of intramammary amoxicillin, frequent milk-out, a combined intramammary amoxicillin, and frequent milk-out treatment versus no treatment. J Dairy Sci 2004;87:583–92.
10. Wilson DJ, Gonzalez RN, Case KL, et al. Comparison of seven antibiotic treatments with no treatment for bacteriologic efficacy against bovine mastitis pathogens. J Dairy Sci 1999;82:1664–70.
11. Guterbock WM, Van Eenennaam AL, Anderson RJ, et al. Efficacy of intramammary antibiotic therapy for treatment of clinical mastitis caused by environmental pathogens. J Dairy Sci 1993;76:3437–44.
12. Hallberg JW, Henke CL, Miller CC. Intramammary antibiotic therapy: to treat or not to treat? Effects on antibiotic therapy on clinical mastitis. In: Proceedings of 26th Annual Meeting of National Mastitis Council, Orlando, FL. National Mastitis Council, Madison (WI), February 20-23, 1987. p. 28–39.
13. Morin DE, Shanks RD, McCoy GC. Comparison of antibiotic administration in conjunction with supportive measures versus supportive measures alone for

treatment of dairy cows with clinical mastitis. J Am Vet Med Assoc 1998;213: 676–84.

14. Schukken YH, Bennett GJ, Zurakowski MJ, et al. Randomized clinical trial to evaluate the efficacy of a 5-day ceftiofur hydrochloride intramammary treatment on nonsevere gram-negative clinical mastitis. J Dairy Sci 2011;94:6203–15.

15. Barkema HW, Schukken YH, Zadoks RN. Invited review: the role of cow, pathogen, and treatment regimen in the therapeutic success of bovine *Staphylococcus aureus* mastitis. J Dairy Sci 2006;89:1877–95.

16. Samson O, Gaudout N, Schmitt E, et al. Use of on-farm data to guide treatment and control mastitis caused by *Streptococcus uberis*. J Dairy Sci 2016;99: 7690–9.

17. Sol J, Sampimon OC, Barkema HE, et al. Factors associated with cure after therapy of clinical mastitis caused by *Staphylococcus aureus*. J Dairy Sci 2000;83: 278–84.

18. Deluyker HA, Michanek P, Wuyts N, et al. Efficacy of Pirlimycin Hydrocloride for treatment of subclinical mastitis in lactating cows. In: Proceedings of the 2nd International Symposium on Mastitis and Milk Quality, Vancouver, BC. National Mastitis Council, Madison (WI) and American Association of Bovine Practitioners, Rome (GA), September 13-15, 2001. p. 224–8.

19. Ziv G, Storper M. Intramuscular treatment of subclinical staphylococcal mastitis in lactating cows with penicillin G, methicillin and their esters. J Vet Pharmacol Ther 1985;8:276–83.

20. Oliver SP, Gillespie BE, Ivey SJ, et al. Efficacy of extended ceftiofur therapy for treatment of naturally occurring subclinical mastitis in lactating dairy cows. J Dairy Sci 2004;87:2393–400.

21. Oliver SP, Almeida RA, Gillespie BE, et al. Extended ceftiofur therapy for treatment of experimentally-induced *Streptococcus uberis* mastitis in lactating dairy cattle. J Dairy Sci 2004;87:3322–9.

22. Gillespie BE, Moorehead H, Dowlen HH, et al. Efficacy of extended pirlimycin therapy for treatment of chronic environmental *Streptococcus* species IMM infections in lactating dairy cows. Vet Ther 2002;3:373–80.

23. Vasquez AK, Nydam DV, Capel MB, et al. Clinical outcome comparison of immediate blanket treatment versus a delayed pathogen-based treatment protocol for clinical mastitis in a New York dairy herd. J Dairy Sci 2017;100:1–12.

24. Vasquez AK, Nydam DV, Capel MB, et al. Randomized noninferiority trial comparing 2 commercial intramammary antibiotics for the treatment of nonsevere clinical mastitis in dairy cows. J Dairy Sci 2016;99:8267–81.

25. Lago A., Tovar C, Zaragoza J, et al. The treatment of only environmental streptococci clinical mastitis cases reduced antibiotic use, days out of the tank, recurrence of clinical mastitis and a tendency to reduce culling. In: Proceedings of 55th Annual Meeting of National Mastitis Council, Glendale, AZ. National Mastitis Council, Madison (WI), January 30 – February 2, 2016. p. 182–3.

26. Tovar C, Pearce D, Lago A, et al. Effect of the selective treatment of Grampositive clinical mastitis cases versus blanket therapy. In: Proceedings of 55th Annual Meeting of National Mastitis Council, Glendale, AZ. National Mastitis Council, Madison (WI), January 30 – February 2, 2016. p. 110–1.

27. Oliveira L, Hulland C, Ruegg PL. Characterization of clinical mastitis occurring in cows on 50 large dairy herds in Wisconsin. J Dairy Sci 2013;96:7538–49.

28. Schukken YH, Zurakowski MJ, Rauch BJ, et al. Noninferiority trial comparing a first-generation cephalosporin with a third-generation cephalosporin in the treatment of nonsevere clinical mastitis in dairy cows. J Dairy Sci 2013;96:1–12.

29. MacDonald KAR. Validation of on farm mastitis pathogen identification systems and determination of the utility of a decision model to target therapy of clinical mastitis during lactation [PhD Thesis]. Charlottetown (PE): University of Prince Edward Island (PE); 2011.

30. Lago A, Godden SM, Bey R, et al. The selective treatment of clinical mastitis based on on-farm culture results: I. Effects on antibiotic use, milk withholding time, and short-term clinical and bacteriological outcomes. J Dairy Sci 2011; 94:4441–56.

31. Pinzón-Sánchez C, Ruegg PL. Risk factors associated with short-term post-treatment outcomes of clinical mastitis. J Dairy Sci 2011;94:3397–410.

32. Bar D, Grohn YT, Bennett G, et al. Effect of repeated episodes of generic clinical mastitis on milk yield in dairy cows. J Dairy Sci 2007;90:4643–53.

33. Olde Riekerink RGM, Barkema HW, Kelton DF, et al. Incidence rate of clinical mastitis on Canadian dairy farms. J Dairy Sci 2008;91:1366–77.

34. Hoe FG, Ruegg PL. Relationship between antimicrobial susceptibility of clinical mastitis pathogens and treatment outcome in cows. J Am Vet Med Assoc 2005;227:1461–8.

35. Kuehn JS, Gorden PJ, Munro D, et al. Bacterial community profiling of milk samples as a means to understand culture-negative bovine clinical mastitis. PLoS One 2013;8:e61959.

36. Rainard P, Riollet C. Innate immunity of the bovine mammary gland. Vet Res 2006; 37:369–400.

37. Hochhalter J, Godden SM, Bey RF, et al. Validation of the Minnesota Easy Culture System II: results from in-lab Bi-plate culture versus standard laboratory culture, and Bi-Plate inter-reader agreement. In: Proceedings of the 39th Annual Convention of the American Association of Bovine Practitioners, St Paul, MN. American Association of Bovine Practitioners, Rome (GA), September 21-23, 2006. p. 298.

38. Lago A. Efficacy of on-farm programs for the diagnosis and selective treatment of clinical and subclinical mastitis in dairy cattle [PhD Thesis]. St Paul (MN): University of Minnesota (MN); 2011.

39. McCarron JL, Keefe GP, McKenna SL, et al. Laboratory evaluation of 3M Petrifilms and University of Minnesota Bi-plates as potential on-farm tests for clinical mastitis. J Dairy Sci 2009;92:2297–305.

40. Royster E, Godden SM, Goulart D, et al. Evaluation of the Minnesota Easy Culture System II Bi-plate and Tri-plate for identification of common mastitis pathogens in milk. J Dairy Sci 2014;97:3648–59.

41. Jones M, Hochhalter J, Bey R, et al. Validation of the Minnesota Easy Culture System II: Results from in-lab Tri-plate culture versus standard laboratory culture, and Tri-plate inter-reader agreement. In: Proceedings of the 39th Annual Convention of the American Association of Bovine Practitioners, St Paul, MN. American Association of Bovine Practitioners, Rome (GA), September 21-23, 2006. p. 299.

42. McCarron JL, Keefe GP, McKenna SL, et al. Evaluation of the University of Minnesota Tri-plate and 3M Petrifilm for the isolation of Staphylococcus aureus and Streptococcus species from clinically mastitic milk samples. J Dairy Sci 2009; 92:5326–33.

43. 3M Microbiology. 3M petrifilm interpretation guide. Saint Paul (MN): 3M Microbiology. 3M; 2005.

44. Mansion-de Vries EM, Knorr N, Paduch JH, et al. A field study evaluation of Petrifilm™ plates as a 24-h rapid diagnostic test for clinical mastitis on a dairy farm. Prev Vet Med 2014;113:620–4.

45. Silva BO, Caraviello DZ, Rodrigues AC, et al. Evaluation of Petrifilm for the isolation of *Staphylococcus aureus* from milk samples. J Dairy Sci 2005;88:3000–8.

46. Ganda EK, Bisinotto RS, Decter DH, et al. Evaluation of an on-farm culture system (Accumast) for fast identification of milk pathogens associated with clinical mastitis in dairy cows. PLoS One 2016;11:e0155314.

47. Ferreira JC, Gomes MS, Bonsaglia ECR, et al. Comparative analysis of four commercial onfarm culture methods to identify bacteria associated with clinical mastitis in dairy cattle. PLoS One 2018;13:e0194211.

48. Griffioen K, Velthuis AG, Lam TJ. On-farm culture results can help to target mastitis treatment decisions. In: Proceedings of 57th Annual Meeting of National Mastitis Council, Tucson, AZ. National Mastitis Council, Madison (WI), 2018. p. 194–5.

49. Erskine RJ, Norby B, Contreras GA, et al. Field evaluation of a dry culture media system to select cows for therapy of clinical mastitis. Proceedings of 54th Annual Meeting of National Mastitis Council, Memphis, TN. National Mastitis Council, Madison (WI), 2015. p. 92–3.

50. Lago A, Godden SM, Bey R, et al. The selective treatment of clinical mastitis based on on-farm culture results: II. Effects on lactation performance, including clinical mastitis recurrence, somatic cell count, milk production, and cow survival. J Dairy Sci 2011;94:4457–67.

51. Steeneveld W, van Werven T, Barkema HW, et al. Cow-specific treatment of clinical mastitis: an economic approach. J Dairy Sci 2011;94:174–88.

52. Pinzón-Sánchez C, Cabrera VE, Ruegg PL. Decision tree analysis of treatment strategies for mild and moderate cases of clinical mastitis occurring in early lactation. J Dairy Sci 2011;94:1873–92.

53. Halasa T. Bioeconomic modeling of intervention against clinical mastitis caused by contagious pathogens. J Dairy Sci 2012;95:5740–9.

54. Down PM, Green MJ, Hudson CD. Rate of transmission: a major determinant of the cost of clinical mastitis. J Dairy Sci 2013;96:6301–14.

55. Lago A, Silva-del-Rio N. Bacteriological culture and California Mastitis Test results of non-clinical quarters from cows with clinical mastitis. Proceedings of 53rd Annual Meeting of National Mastitis Council, Fort Worth, TX. National Mastitis Council, Madison (WI), 2014. p. 203–4.

56. Lago A, Silva-del-Rio N, Blanc C. Preliminary evaluation of the use of bacteriological culture after the treatment of clinical mastitis with antibiotics. Proceedings of 52nd Annual Meeting of National Mastitis Council, San Diego, CA. National Mastitis Council, Madison (WI), 2013. p. 157.

57. Minnesota easy culture system II user's manual. Saint Paul (MN): University of Minnesota; 2013.

Making Antibiotic Treatment Decisions for Clinical Mastitis

Pamela L. Ruegg, DVM, MPVM

KEYWORDS

- Mastitis • Antibiotics • Udder health • Treatment • Milk quality

KEY POINTS

- Mastitis is diagnosed based on detection of inflammation, but inflammation does not always indicate continued presence of active bacterial infection.
- Only about one-third of cases of nonsevere clinical mastitis occurring on many modern dairy farms will benefit from use of antibiotics.
- Antibiotic therapy is indicated when the spontaneous cure is significantly less than the expected treatment cure rate and the case is caused by a pathogen that is susceptible to approved intramammary antibiotics.
- The medical history of the cow should be assessed before giving antibiotics to determine if the cow is a good candidate for antibiotic therapy.
- It is not possible for farmers or veterinarians to determine the short-term efficacy of antibiotic treatments based on clinical outcomes.

INTRODUCTION

Mastitis is an infectious disease that is diagnosed based on observation of an inflammatory response that occurs after an intramammary infection (IMI). Most cases are caused by bacteria and vary in presentation depending on the characteristics of the pathogen and the ability of the cow to mount a rapid and effective immune response. When inflammation results in visible abnormalities of milk, the mammary gland, or the cow, the infection is usually considered to be a case of clinical mastitis (CM) and the abnormal milk must be discarded. On most farms, greater than 85% of cases of CM present with only mild (abnormal milk) or moderate (local signs, such as swollen udder) signs and are classified as nonsevere.[1] Although severe cases (with generalized signs, such as fever, anorexia, distress, and so forth) are medical emergencies and should immediately be treated using protocols developed with veterinary input, in North America most treatments of nonsevere CM are performed by farm workers without

Department of Animal Science, Michigan State University, 474 South Shaw Lane, East Lansing, MI 48864, USA
E-mail address: plruegg@msu.edu

Vet Clin Food Anim 34 (2018) 413–425
https://doi.org/10.1016/j.cvfa.2018.06.002
0749-0720/18/© 2018 Elsevier Inc. All rights reserved.

vetfood.theclinics.com

veterinary supervision. Nonsevere CM is a common disease, and treatment of this condition is the most common reason that antibiotics[a] are given to mature dairy cows.[2,3]

Use of antimicrobials to treat farm animals is increasingly scrutinized and must be justified as necessary to maintain animal well-being.[4] Appropriate use of antibiotics for the treatment of nonsevere CM is based on understanding the etiology, review of the cow's medical history and application of well-recognized therapeutic principles to select among approved antibiotics.[5,6] Increased involvement of veterinarians in development of mastitis treatment protocols is needed to ensure appropriate usage. On many farms, almost all mastitis is treated using antibiotics[1] but not all cases of nonsevere CM will benefit from antimicrobial therapy and protocols used to treat these cases should include alternatives strategies for managing those cases.[6] The purpose of this article is to review use of antimicrobials for treatment of nonsevere CM to help veterinarians develop protocols that ensure responsible usage.

HISTORICAL DEVELOPMENT OF TREATMENT PROTOCOLS

In 1947, Murphy[7] confirmed that mastitis was a result of invasion of an organism followed by establishment of IMI and development of inflammation. In those years, almost all bovine mastitis was caused by *Streptococcus agalactiae* and *Staphylococcus aureus* and most treatment protocols were originally developed to combat those pathogens. The high prevalence and desire to eradicate *S agalactiae* was a significant historical factor that established routine use of intramammary antibiotics for treatment of CM and for treatment of dry cows.[8] As these organisms were controlled in the 1980s, researchers recognized that CM caused by coliform bacteria was becoming more prevalent (even in herds with a low somatic cell count [SCC]) and recognized that many of these cases spontaneously resolved without use of antimicrobials.[9–12] The continued emphasis on treatment of pathogens that are no longer common on many dairy farms is apparent when reviewing label claims of intramammary antibiotics sold in the United States and Canada. Of intramammary antibiotics sold in these countries, efficacy against *S aureus* and *S agalactiae* is the primary efficacy claim for 7 of the 8 approved products. As causes of CM have changed it is imperative for veterinarians to reexamine recommendations for management of nonsevere CM. Continued use of treatment protocols that were developed in an era that had different distributions of pathogens is difficult to justify.

ETIOLOGY OF CLINICAL MASTITIS ON MODERN DAIRY FARMS

As dairy farms have enlarged and become more intensively managed, the distribution of pathogens recovered from cases of CM has become more diverse and on most farms is dominated by opportunistic environmental organisms (**Fig. 1**). Based on herd surveys conducted in many countries,[1,13–18] the most common outcome of culturing milk collected from cases of CM is usually no microbial growth (about 30%), followed by either coliforms (about 30% in intensively managed cows) or environmental streptococci (up to 45% in extensively managed cows in New Zealand). The proportion of cases caused by *S aureus* is highly variable, ranging from 3% in large

---

[a] The terms *antimicrobial* and *antibiotic* are used interchangeably in this article but are not synonymous. In technical terms, *antibiotics* refers only to substances of microbial origin (such as penicillin) that are active against other microbes, whereas *antimicrobial* refers to any substance (including synthetic compounds) that destroys microbes.

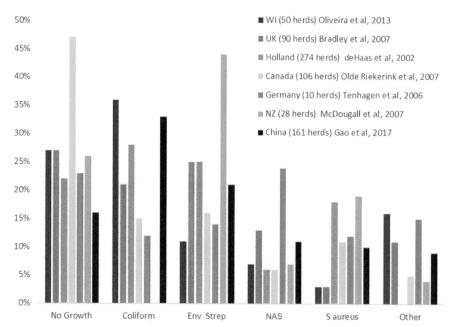

Fig. 1. Results of studies that describe the distribution of bacteria recovered from milk of cows with CM in modern-dairy herds in selected countries. NAS, non-aureus staphylcocci; Env Strep, environmental streptococci.

herds in Wisconsin[1] to 11% in a Canadian national survey[8,19] and 19% in New Zealand,[20] but is usually more prevalent in studies that include smaller herds, extensive management systems, or emerging dairy regions. Overall, about 5% and 7% of cases of CM were caused by other pathogens or the non-aureus staphylococci (NAS), respectively. When data from these studies (see **Fig. 1**) are combined, the weighted average distribution of causes for CM are no growth (26%), environmental streptococci (22%), coliform bacteria (26%), *S aureus* (12%), non-aureus staphylococci (NAS) (8%), and other pathogens (6%). Recognition of the diversity of agents and the proportion of culture-negative results is important to ensure responsible use of antibiotics. On individual farms, the cost-effectiveness of antimicrobial therapy for the treatment of nonsevere CM depends highly on the use of antimicrobials that effectively target predominant etiologic agents. The unnecesary cost of giving intramammary (IMM) antibiotics to patients that are not expected to benefit can be substantial (**Fig. 2**). The scenario in **Fig. 2** is based on nonspecific treatment of 400 patients with CM using a very-low-cost, short-duration treatment (2 tubes of intramammary antibiotics that cost $3.25 each). Of approximately $3000 in annual costs of product, less than $1000 can be expected to result in a bacteriologic cure in excess of an expected spontaneous cure and failure to cure (due to intrinsic resistance). Veterinarians are encouraged to work with dairy producers to increase the use of selective treatment protocols, as symptomatic treatment of nonsevere CM without knowledge of etiology results in overuse and economically nonsustainable use of antibiotics.

Over time, the number of milk samples collected from cases of CM that are culture negative has increased.[21] Reasons that milk samples from mastitis cases are culture negative varies based on etiology and case presentation. Cows with chronic

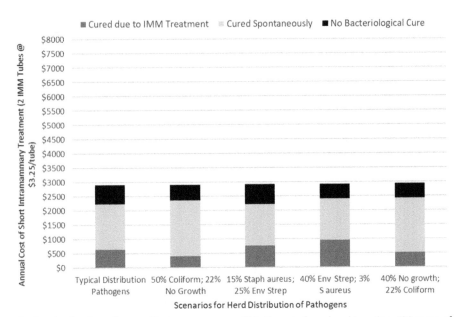

Fig. 2. Distribution of annual intramammary antibiotic costs for a herd treating 400 cases of CM per year using 2 intramammary antibiotic tubes at $3.25 per tube for all cases of CM, regardless of etiology. Env Strep, environmental streptococci.

subclinical mastitis (defined as normal-appearing milk but a long history of high SCC) have strong evidence of on-going failed inflammation that is, most likely the result of persistent IMI. These cases are often false negatives because the large inflammatory response has successfully reduced the number of organisms to less than the normal detection limit (about 100 colony-forming units per milliliter in most mastitis laboratories). Repeated culturing of quarter-milk samples may help arrive at a diagnosis for some of these cases. In contrast, many mild and moderate cases of CM are caused by opportunistic pathogens that have been successfully eliminated by a localized immune response before detection of inflammation. The clinical signs of abnormal milk are detected after the initial immune response, and about 75% to 85% of these cases may be spontaneously cured before detection. Unfortunately, the only way to determine if the clinical signs of nonsevere CM are accompanied by active infection (and thus will benefit from antimicrobial therapy) is to perform microbiological analysis. In some regions, increasingly diverse causes recovered from cases of CM have stimulated the use of selective treatment protocols that limit antibiotic usage to those caused by pathogens that require antimicrobial therapy to improve bacterial clearance.[22,23] Although these are good steps forward, additional cost-effective and easily implemented diagnostic tools are needed to further enhance implementation of these strategies.

ASSESSING PROGNOSIS

Mastitis is caused by a diverse group of bacteria that vary among farms and the probability of achieving a successful outcome is highly influenced by the characteristics of individual pathogens. Depending on virulence factors, organisms infect different sites within the mammary gland, have differing abilities to cause systemic signs, and vary in expected duration of subclinical phases of infection and expectations for spontaneous bacteriologic cure. Estimates of bacteriologic cure after treatment of CM caused by gram-positive pathogens have ranged from 25% (*S aureus*) to about 65% to 70% (environmental streptococci species and NAS).[24] In contrast, bacteriologic cure of mastitis caused by *Escherichia coli* often exceed 75%.[25] On most farms, about 25% to 40% of clinical cases are microbiologically negative when detected; clinical outcomes of these cases are usually positive.[24,26]

On larger US farms, *E coli* is a common cause of mastitis; about two-thirds of cases caused by this organism present with symptoms that are localized to the udder.[1] The rate of spontaneous cure for these mild infections is quite high because the point of infection within the udder is generally superficial mucosal surfaces of the mammary gland cisterns and ducts. On other farms, mastitis is frequently caused by environmental streptococci species, and spontaneous bacteriologic cure rates of these organisms vary among species with some researchers reporting higher rates for *Streptococcus dysgalactiae* as compared with *Streptococcus uberis*.[27] Environmental streptococci species often respond well to intramammary (IMM) antimicrobial therapy but have a low spontaneous cure rate and high rate of recurrence when antimicrobials are not administered. Determination of the etiology of IMI through the use of rapid farm or veterinary clinic-based culturing programs can considerably reduce unnecessary antimicrobial usage while still resulting in satisfactory treatment outcomes.

ASSESSING OUTCOMES

Based on assessment of clinical signs, it is extremely difficult for farm workers or veterinary practitioners to determine if antimicrobial therapy has been effective. The inability of clinical signs to predict bacterial clearance was first noted in 1938 when a researcher administered massive doses of sulfanilamide but failed to achieve therapeutic concentrations in either blood or milk. The researcher noted that "treatment with sulfanilamide was successful in restoring normal flow and normal appearance of milk...but it did not eliminate the streptococci from the udder, nor prevent later acute attacks."[28] This comment is the first indication that clinical impressions are often misleading in determining the efficacy of antimicrobial compounds and also illustrate the difficulty of separating the occurrence of inflammation from active IMI.

Judgements about efficacy of mastitis treatments are generally based on perceptions of how the products performed in the past and are rarely based on objective evaluation of appropriate data.[29] Occurrence of abnormal milk is the most obvious sign of CM, and many farmers assess treatments based on the number of days that milk is discarded. However, this outcome has little variation[24] and is greatly influenced by factors other than treatment (especially etiology; FUENZALIDA ADSA 2017).[30] On some dairy farms, the duration of treatment or choice of drug is based on the appearance of abnormal milk. An abnormal appearance of milk is a nonspecific sign of inflammation that is not always associated with continued IMI and is not predictive of the etiology.

Most approved IMM drugs are active against organisms that are rapidly dividing, and there is no evidence that changing among drugs with similar spectrums of activity or extending duration based on continued appearance of abnormal milk will result in improved clinical or bacteriologic outcomes. Neither duration of treatment nor choice of drug should be based solely on appearance of milk or on indirect indicators, such as California Mastitis Test or quarter-level SCC values. With or without treatment or bacterial clearance, about 85% of cows affected with nonsevere CM caused by coliform bacteria will have normal appearing milk by day 7 (Fuenzalida and Ruegg, personal communication, 2018). Regardless of etiology, after initial therapy, if milk remains abnormal for more than 6 or 7 days, before administration of another antibiotic, every attempt should be made to determine the etiology of the infection as it is unlikely that switching among drugs with similar spectrums will improve clinical outcomes.

The purpose of antibiotic treatment is to enhance clearance of bacterial pathogens, and efficacy of products is usually initially evaluated based on estimates of the rate of bacteriologic cure. Bacteriologic cure is assessed by comparison of recovery of bacteria from milk samples collected at detection of the cases and subsequently at various intervals after treatment is completed. However, bacteriologic cure also occurs spontaneously and expected rates of spontaneous bacteriologic cure vary widely among pathogens (**Table 1**). The greatest contrast is between expectations of spontaneous bacteriologic cure of IMI caused by S aureus (close to zero) and CM caused by E coli (about 90%[25].) Additionally, limited efficacy of antibiotic therapy is well documented for IMI caused by S aureus[31,32]; some pathogens (such as yeast, Prototheca zopfii, Mycoplasma spp, and others) are intrinsically resistant to all approved antimicrobial drugs. It is important to note that even with highly efficacious drugs, the benefit of antimicrobial therapy is only for cases that are not expected to achieve spontaneous bacteriological cure; thus, the value of antibiotic therapy decreases for cases caused by E coli or other pathogens with high rates of spontaneous cure.

GUIDELINES FOR APPROPRIATE USE OF ANTIBIOTICS

Guidelines for appropriate use of antibiotics have been developed[33] and should be applied to mastitis treatments. The most significant guidelines are that *antibiotic usage should involve veterinary guidance and extralabel use should be avoided when on-label use is a possibility*. Veterinarians and producers in the United States should be aware of label indications and claims of efficacy and recognize that extralabel treatments occur when systemic antibiotics are administered or when the dosing regimen of intramammary products is altered from that described on the label. Deviations from label guidelines are common for mastitis treatment and may be justifiable for some drugs but must be done under veterinary supervision. Extralabel use of parenteral antibiotics to treat mastitis is not unusual[3,24,34,35] but should be restricted to justifiable cases, such as cows affected with severe mastitis.

Table 1
Estimated rate of spontaneous bacteriologic cure by pathogen from selected studies

Cause	Spontaneous Bacteriologic Cure (%)	Sources
S aureus	0–11	Oliver et al,[37] 2004; Deluyker et al,[48] 1999; Gillespie et al,[49] 2002
Env streptococci species	28–30	Deluyker et al,[48] 1999; Hoe & Ruegg,[50] 2005; Morin and Constable,[51] 1998
Non-aureus staphylococci (NAS)	44–66	Oliver et al,[37] 2004; Deluyker et al,[48] 1999; Apparao et al,[52] 2009
E coli	80–95	Fuenzalida & Ruegg, personal communication; Lago et al,[22] 2011; Suojala et al,[53] 2010
Klebsiella spp	25–60	Lago et al,[22] 2011; Fuenzalida & Ruegg, personal communication, 2018
No growth	75–85	Fuenzalida & Ruegg, personal communication, 2018

Appropriate usage guidelines[33] also specify that *antibiotics should only be used when there is a reasonable likelihood that a bacterial infection that is sensitive to the proposed antibiotic is present.* Given that 20% to 40% of CM cases are culture negative, this criterion is often not achieved; alternative ways to manage these case should be considered. Antibiotics should not be used for cows that are unlikely to benefit and selective treatment based on on-farm or veterinary clinic laboratories is advised. Practitioners should also ensure that antimicrobials are not given to cows affected with nonsevere CM caused by a refractory pathogen, such as *Mycoplasma bovis*, *S aureus*, *Prototheca*, and *Serratia*. When antibiotics are not likely to be effective, abnormal milk should be discarded until it returns to normal (usually about 4–6 days); frequent observation of the cow's behavior and symptoms (watchful waiting) is recommended to detect the rare instances when severity progresses.

Depending on intrinsic bacterial susceptibility, antibiotics are classified as either narrow or broad spectrum. Narrow-spectrum drugs are usually active against either gram-positive or gram-negative bacteria, whereas broad-spectrum drugs have activity against both types of organisms. The World Health Organization has classified antibiotics based on their importance for treating human illnesses,[36] and responsible usage guidelines suggest that *narrow spectrum antibiotics that are less critical for treating human illnesses should be used as a first choice.*[33] Most IMM products available in the United States are not high-priority drugs for treatment of human illnesses and only ceftiofur (a third-generation cephalosporin) is listed as both high priority and critically important for human use.[36] Most approved IMM products are considered narrow spectrum, and the use of the broader-spectrum IMM drugs should be reserved for cases that will benefit.

Responsible usage guidelines propose that *antibiotics should be used for as short a duration as possible.* The appropriate duration of antibiotic treatment of CM is not well defined and varies depending on the etiology. Some pathogens preferentially infect superficial mucosal surfaces, whereas other pathogens have the ability to deeply infiltrate mammary gland secretory tissue. There is limited evidence that extended-duration antibiotic therapy increases the bacterial cure of invasive pathogens (such as *S aureus* and some environmental streptococci species).[37,38] However, no research has indicated that extended-duration therapy improves clinical outcomes of mastitis caused by noninvasive pathogens (such as NAS or most *E coli*). The use of extended-duration therapy to treat these types of pathogens significantly increases costs without improving economic outcomes.[39] It is important to note that when extended IMM therapy is considered, veterinarians need to assess the ability of farm workers to perform aseptic infusions, as extended IMM treatment is associated with an increased risk of infection from opportunistic pathogens.

Appropriate usage guidelines infer that the cow is healthy enough to respond, and veterinarians should ensure that treatment protocols include the review of the cow's medical history before making a decision to give antibiotics. The purpose of antibiotic therapy is to assist the immune response, and many characteristics of the cow are known to influence the probability of a successful immune response.[40] Characteristics related to a healthy immune response include age, stage of lactation, negative energy balance, history of previous treatments, and environmental factors (such as heat stress). Older cattle ($\geq$third parity) often have poorer responses to treatment as compared with younger cattle.[14,20,41] A history of chronically increased SCC is also associated with a poorer prognosis after mastitis therapy.[42,43] Cows in the immediate postpartum period are known to be immunosuppressed, and heat stress can reduce the ability of the cow to respond to an IMI.[44] Before administration of antibiotics, the herd-health manager should assess if the cow has risk factors that indicate antibiotics may be beneficial. For example, short-duration IMM antibiotics may be considered for CM occurring in valuable older cows that have nonsevere gram-negative mastitis in the immediate postpartum period. Conversely, watchful waiting may be considered for CM occurring in older cows that have a long history of repeated nonsevere cases.

DETERMINING THE APPROPRIATE TREATMENT

Surveys of dairy producers indicate that IMM antibiotics are used to treat most cases of mastitis.[3,24,29] In the United States, there are 7 approved IMMs; No systemically administered antibiotics are approved for treatment of mastitis and IMM antibiotics should be used as the first choice for treatment of nonsevere CM. Approved IMM products have pharmacologic characteristics that ensure a sufficient concentration of the drug (or active metabolite) will be present in the udder during the approved dosing interval to kill or restrict growth of the organisms listed on the product label. Almost all approved IMM antibiotics are labeled for treatment of *Streptococci* and *Staphylococci,* and 2 products include label claims for *E coli*. No products have claims for the treatment of mastitis caused by *Klebsiella spp*; but when treatment of mastitis caused by this organism is attempted, extralabel IMM administration of a drug with known gram-negative activity is recommended. Little to no research exists to support the efficacy claims for other organisms, and the lack of efficacy data makes it very difficult to justify the use of antibiotics for the treatment of mastitis caused by many pathogens.

Research has shown that extralabel use of systemic antibiotics (such as injectable ceftiofur) is beneficial for the treatment of septicemia that occurs in many cows affected with severe mastitis.[45,46] However, no benefit has been demonstrated when ceftiofur was administered systemically to cows affected with nonsevere CM.[47] Systemic administration of most antibiotics that are allowed under extralabel guidelines is not likely to result in therapeutic concentrations in the udder, and this use is not recommended for the treatment of nonsevere CM. As most mastitis treatments are administered simply based on observation of inflammation (without knowledge of the pathogen), most systemic treatments are difficult to justify both medically and to consumers.

MAKING TREATMENT DECISIONS FOR NONSEVERE CLINICAL MASTITIS

The decision to use an antibiotic for the treatment of nonsevere CM should be based on a reasonable expectation that an active bacterial infection is occurring in a cow who has a reasonable probability of responding to treatment using an antimicrobial with an appropriate spectrum of activity and that the use of the antibiotic will result in clinical outcomes that exceed expectations if antimicrobials are not administered.

The initial decision for nonsevere cases is to identify cows that may not be responsive to antibiotic therapy and using watchful waiting or other options for managing these cases. Watchful waiting refers to simply monitoring the cow, discarding her milk and waiting for the inflammation to subsist, which usually occurs within about 4 to 6 days.[22,24,26] After the milk returns to normal, the cow can be returned to the milking herd; but segregation in a group of cows with high SCC is often recommended. Permanent dry off of the affected quarter is an option for quarters that have received multiple antibiotic treatments. Culling should be the first choice for cows that are diagnosed with *Mycoplasma bovis* and most cows infected with *S aureus*.

After assessing the cow, determination of etiology is recommended. Based on the typical distribution of pathogens that cause CM (see **Fig. 1**), if antibiotics are administered to all cases based on clinical signs only, their benefits are reduced. Using reported values for pathogen-specific rates of spontaneous cure (see **Table 1**) and assumptions about treatment efficacy for various pathogens (**Table 2**), the overall proportion of cases that can be expected to benefit from nonspecific antibiotic therapy ranges from about 20% to 33% (see **Table 2**). Thus, approximately two-thirds of antibiotic treatments given by farmers who administer antibiotics to all cases of nonsevere CM (without knowledge of etiology) are of no or limited benefit to the cow. When pathogen-specific treatments are not feasible, only some cows will benefit from antibiotics and even fewer will benefit from extended-duration therapy; in this instance, the best economic decision is to treat for a short duration using an IMM antibiotic.[39] When short-duration therapy is used, it is important to recognize that treatment will usually be completed before milk returns to normal appearance.

When possible, pathogen-specific treatment programs are preferable. In most selective treatment protocols, no antibiotic treatment is given until the preliminary results of the culture are known (generally 24 hours), whereas in other protocols, treatment is initiated after the milk sample is collected and results of preliminary cultures are used to modify therapy. The concept of culture-based treatment is to administer antibiotics only for cases that have active (culture positive) infections caused by pathogens (usually gram positive) that are likely to be sensitive to approved IMM antibiotics. For cases with no microbial growth or gram-negative growth, milk is simply discarded until it returns to normal or antiinflammatories may be given if indicated (some moderate

Table 2
Proportion of nonsevere cases of clinical mastitis that would be expected to achieve bacteriologic cure from routine IMM antibiotic therapy used without knowledge of etiology

Actual Cause	A. Proportion of Cases[a] (%)	B. Assumed Rate of Spontaneous Bacterial Cure (%)	C. Scenario 1: Some Benefit of Antibiotic (%)	D. Scenario 2: Highly Efficacious Antibiotic[c] (%)	A × (1 − B) × C Scenario 1 (%)	A × (1 − B) × D Scenario 2 (%)
No growth	26	85	15	50	0.59	1.95
Coliforms	26	75	25	50	1.63	3.25
Env streptococci	22	20	80	95	14.08	16.72
NAS	8	60	40	80	1.28	2.56
S aureus	12	10	25	60	2.70	6.48
Others	6	50	5	20	0.15	0.60
Proportion of cases benefiting from antibiotic usage (%):					20.4	31.6
Proportion of treated cases receiving no benefit from antibiotics (%):				79.6	68.4	

Columns C and D are grouped under "Assumed Efficacy of IMM Treatment[b]"; the last two columns under "Proportion of Total Cases Benefiting from Antibiotic Usage[d]".

Abbreviation: Env, environmental.
[a] Weighted average of studies included in **Fig. 1**.
[b] Proportion of cases *in excess of spontaneous cures* that would result in bacteriologic cure due to antibiotic therapy.
[c] Assumes reduced rate of spontaneous cure and increased efficacy of antibiotic.
[d] Calculated as proportion of cases × (1−spontaneous cure) × assumed efficacy of IMM treatment.

cases). For more information on the development of culture programs please see Alfonso Lago and Sandra M. Godden's article, "Use of Rapid Culture Systems to Guide Etiology-Based Clinical Mastitis Treatment Decisions," in this issue.

When nonantibiotic treatment strategies are used, we are assuming that the immune response will be effective in clearing the infection. Thus, it is essential for veterinarians to ensure that the medical history of the cow is assessed before withholding antibiotics. When cows have conditions that result in immune suppression, (immediate postpartum period, severe negative energy balance, concurrent disease, and so forth) or if a culture-negative case or gram-negative case is preceded by a long period of increased SCC (indicating that the cow's immune system has not been successful in eliminating the pathogen), short-duration IMM therapy may be considered.

SUMMARY

Appropriate use of antimicrobials on dairy farms contributes to improving animal well-being and dairy farm sustainability but it is important for veterinarians to recognize that many cases of nonsevere CM will not benefit from antimicrobial therapy. Mastitis is caused by a diverse group of bacterial pathogens with differing distributions among farms. In intensively managed herds, many cases of CM are culture-negative when detected or are caused by pathogens with high rates of spontaneous cure. In such herds, when treatments are administered without knowledge of etiology, most antimicrobial treatments are likely to be unnecessary. There is considerable opportunity for veterinarians to improve antimicrobial usage on dairy farms by encouraging farmers to adopt culture-based treatment protocols that limit antimicrobial usage to cases that will benefit. When this option is not feasible, farmers should be encouraged to review the medical history of the cow before treatment and, when antimicrobial use is warranted, initiate therapy using a narrow-spectrum drug for a short duration.

REFERENCES

1. Oliveira L, Hulland C, Ruegg PL. Characterization of clinical mastitis occurring in cows on 50 large dairy herds in Wisconsin. J Dairy Sci 2013;96(12):7538–49.
2. Saini V, McClure JT, Leger D, et al. Antimicrobial use on Canadian dairy farms. J Dairy Sci 2012;95(3):1209–21.
3. Pol M, Ruegg PL. Treatment practices and quantification of antimicrobial drug usage in conventional and organic dairy farms in Wisconsin. J Dairy Sci 2007;90(1):249–61.
4. Ruegg PL. Minimizing development of antimicrobial resistance on dairy farms through appropriate use of antibiotics for treatment of mastitis. In: Van Belzen N, editor. Achieving sustainable production of cow's milk, vol. 2. Belgium: Burleigh Dodds; 2017. p. 117–33.
5. Ruegg PL. Antibiotic treatments for bovine mastitis: who, what, when, how and why? Paper presented at: Ann. Meeting Am. Assoc. Bov. Pract, Milwaukee, WI, September 19-21, 2013.
6. Ruegg PL. Practical approaches to mastitis therapy on large dairy herds. In: Hogan J, editor. Large dairy herd management. 3rd edition. Champaign (IL): Am. Dairy Sci. Assoc.; 2017.
7. Murphy JM. The genesis of bovine udder infection and mastitis; the occurrence of streptococcal infection in a cow population during a seven-year period and its relationship to age. Am J Vet Res 1947;8(26):29–42.
8. Ruegg PL. A 100-year review: mastitis detection, management, and prevention. J Dairy Sci 2017;100(12):10381–97.

9. Hogan JS, Smith KL, Hoblet KH, et al. Field survey of clinical mastitis in low somatic cell count herds. J Dairy Sci 1989;72(6):1547–56.

10. Smith KL, Todhunter DA, Schoenberger PS. Environmental mastitis: cause, prevalence, prevention. J Dairy Sci 1985;68(6):1531–53.

11. Pyorala S. Therapeutic treatment of the acute form of the clinical mastitis - compilatory account. Magy Allatorvosok Lapja 1994;49(9):536–41.

12. Pyorala S, Kaartinen L, Kack H, et al. Efficacy of two therapy regimens for treatment of experimentally induced Escherichia coli mastitis in cows. J Dairy Sci 1994;77(2):453–61.

13. Riekerink RGMO, Barkema HW, Stryhn H. The effect of season on somatic cell count and the incidence of clinical mastitis. J Dairy Sci 2007;90(4):1704–15.

14. McDougall S, Agnew KE, Cursons R, et al. Parenteral treatment of clinical mastitis with tylosin base or penethamate hydriodide in dairy cattle. J Dairy Sci 2007; 90(2):779–89.

15. Bradley AJ, Leach KA, Breen JE, et al. Survey of the incidence and aetiology of mastitis on dairy farms in England and Wales. Vet Rec 2007;160(8):253–7.

16. de Haas Y, Barkema HW, Veerkamp RF. The effect of pathogen-specific clinical mastitis on the lactation curve for somatic cell count. J Dairy Sci 2002;85(5): 1314–23.

17. Gao J, Barkema HW, Zhang L, et al. Incidence of clinical mastitis and distribution of pathogens on large Chinese dairy farms. J Dairy Sci 2017;100(6):4797–806.

18. Tenhagen BA, Koster G, Wallmann J, et al. Prevalence of mastitis pathogens and their resistance against antimicrobial agents in dairy cows in Brandenburg, Germany. J Dairy Sci 2006;89(7):2542–51.

19. Olde Riekerink RGM, Barkema HW, Kelton DF, et al. Incidence rate of clinical mastitis on Canadian dairy farms. J Dairy Sci 2008;91(4):1366–77.

20. McDougall S, Arthur DG, Bryan MA, et al. Clinical and bacteriological response to treatment of clinical mastitis with one of three intramammary antibiotics. N Z Vet J 2007;55(4):161–70.

21. Makovec JA, Ruegg PL. Results of milk samples submitted for microbiological examination in Wisconsin from 1994 to 2001. J Dairy Sci 2003;86(11):3466–72.

22. Lago A, Godden SM, Bey R, et al. The selective treatment of clinical mastitis based on on-farm culture results: I. Effects on antibiotic use, milk withholding time, and short-term clinical and bacteriological outcomes. J Dairy Sci 2011; 94(9):4441–56.

23. Lago A, Godden SM, Bey R, et al. The selective treatment of clinical mastitis based on on-farm culture results: II. Effects on lactation performance, including clinical mastitis recurrence, somatic cell count, milk production, and cow survival. J Dairy Sci 2011;94(9):4457–67.

24. Oliveira L, Ruegg PL. Treatments of clinical mastitis occurring in cows on 51 large dairy herds in Wisconsin. J Dairy Sci 2014;97(9):5426–36.

25. Suojala L, Kaartinen L, Pyorala S. Treatment for bovine Escherichia coli mastitis - an evidence-based approach. J Vet Pharmacol Ther 2013;36(6):521–31.

26. Fuenzalida MJ, Baumberger C, Ruegg PL. Preliminary results of a clinical trial evaluating effects of treatment of culture negative cases of clinical mastitis on SCC and milk production. Paper presented at: National Mastitis Council. Phoenix, AZ, Jan 31–Feb 2, 2016.

27. Vasquez AK, Nydam DV, Capel MB, et al. Randomized noninferiority trial comparing 2 commercial intramammary antibiotics for the treatment of nonsevere clinical mastitis in dairy cows. J Dairy Sci 2016;99(10):8267–81.

28. Gildow EM, Fourt DL, Shaw AO. Sulfanilamide in the Treatment of Streptococcic Mastitis. J Dairy Sci 1938;21(12):759–66.
29. USDA. Dairy 2007, part III: reference of dairy cattle health and management practices in the United States, 2007. Fort Collins (CO): USDA-APHIS-VS, CEAH; 2008.
30. Fuenzalida MJ, Ruegg PL. Quarter somatic cell count of culture negative and Gram-negative cases of non-severe clinical mastitis enrolled in negatively controlled randomized clinical trials. J Dairy Sci 2017;100:232.
31. Barkema HW, Schukken YH, Zadoks RN. Invited review: the role of cow, pathogen, and treatment regimen in the therapeutic success of bovine Staphylococcus aureus mastitis. J Dairy Sci 2006;89(6):1877–95.
32. Philpot WN. Role of therapy in mastitis control. J Dairy Sci 1969;52(5):708–13.
33. Weese JS, Page SW, Prescott JF. Antimicrobial stewardship in animals. In: Giguere S, Prescott JF, Dowling PM, editors. Antimicrobial therapy. Ames (IA): Wiley Blackwell; 2013. p. 117–33.
34. Raymond MJ, Wohrle RD, Call DR. Assessment and promotion of judicious antibiotic use on dairy farms in Washington state. J Dairy Sci 2006;89(8):3228–40.
35. USDA. Dairy 2007, part V: changes in dairy cattle health and management practices in the United States, 1996–2007. Fort Collins (CO): USDA, CEAS, NAHMS; 2009.
36. Anonymous. Critically important antimicrobials for human health - 3rd rev. 2012:32. Available at: http://apps.who.int/iris/bitstream/10665/77376/1/9789241504485_eng.pdf. Accessed January 20, 2016.
37. Oliver SP, Almeida RA, Gillespie BE, et al. Extended ceftiofur therapy for treatment of experimentally-induced Streptococcus uberis mastitis in lactating dairy cattle. J Dairy Sci 2004;87(10):3322–9.
38. Oliver SP, Gillespie BE, Headrick SJ, et al. Efficacy of extended ceftiofur intramammary therapy for treatment of subclinical mastitis in lactating dairy cows. J Dairy Sci 2004;87(8):2393–400.
39. Pinzon-Sanchez C, Cabrera VE, Ruegg PL. Decision tree analysis of treatment strategies for mild and moderate cases of clinical mastitis occurring in early lactation. J Dairy Sci 2011;94(4):1873–92.
40. Burvenich C, Van Merris V, Mehrzad J, et al. Severity of E. coli mastitis is mainly determined by cow factors. Vet Res 2003;34(5):521–64.
41. Hektoen L, Odegaard SA, Loken T, et al. Evaluation of stratification factors and score-scales in clinical trials of treatment of clinical mastitis in dairy cows. J Vet Med A Physiol Pathol Clin Med 2004;51(4):196–202.
42. Bradley AJ, Green MJ. Factors affecting cure when treating bovine clinical mastitis with cephalosporin-based intramammary preparations. J Dairy Sci 2009;92(5):1941–53.
43. Pinzon-Sanchez C, Ruegg PL. Risk factors associated with short-term post-treatment outcomes of clinical mastitis. J Dairy Sci 2011;94(7):3397–410.
44. do Amaral BC, Connor EE, Tao S, et al. Heat stress abatement during the dry period influences metabolic gene expression and improves immune status in the transition period of dairy cows. J Dairy Sci 2011;94(1):86–96.
45. Erskine RJ, Bartlett PC, VanLente JL, et al. Efficacy of systemic ceftiofur as a therapy for severe clinical mastitis in dairy cattle. J Dairy Sci 2002;85(10):2571–5.
46. Wenz JR, Barrington GM, Garry FB, et al. Bacteremia associated with naturally occurring acute coliform mastitis in dairy cows. J Am Vet Med Assoc 2001; 219(7):976–81.

47. Wenz JR, Garry FB, Lombard JE, et al. Efficacy of parenteral ceftiofur for treatment of systemically mild clinical mastitis in dairy cattle. J Dairy Sci 2005; 88(10):3496–9.
48. Deluyker HA, Chester ST, Van Oye SN. A multilocation clinical trial in lactating dairy cows affected with clinical mastitis to compare the efficacy of treatment with intramammary infusions of a lincomycin/neomycin combination with an ampicillin/cloxacillin combination. J Vet Pharmacol Ther 1999;22(4):274–82.
49. Gillespie BE, Moorehead H, Lunn P, et al. Efficacy of extended pirlimycin hydrochloride therapy for treatment of environmental Streptococcus spp and Staphylococcus aureus intramammary infections in lactating dairy cows. Vet Ther 2002; 3(4):373–80.
50. Hoe FG, Ruegg PL. Relationship between antimicrobial susceptibility of clinical mastitis pathogens and treatment outcome in cows. J Am Vet Med Assoc 2005;227(9):1461–8.
51. Morin DE, Constable PD. Characteristics of dairy cows during episodes of bacteriologically negative clinical mastitis or mastitis caused by Corynebacterium spp. J Am Vet Med Assoc 1998;213(6):855–61.
52. Apparao D, Oliveira L, Ruegg PL. Relationship between results of in vitro susceptibility tests and outcomes following treatment with pirlimycin hydrochloride in cows with subclinical mastitis associated with gram-positive pathogens. J Am Vet Med Assoc 2009;234(11):1437–46.
53. Suojala L, Simojoki H, Mustonen K, et al. Efficacy of enrofloxacin in the treatment of naturally occurring acute clinical Escherichia coli mastitis. J Dairy Sci 2010; 93(5):1960–9.

Understanding the Milk Microbiota

Stephanie A. Metzger, PhD[a,b], Laura L. Hernandez, PhD[a], Garret Suen, PhD[c], Pamela L. Ruegg, DVM, MPVM[d],*

KEYWORDS

- Milk microbiota • Milk microbiome • Mastitis

KEY POINTS

- The milk microbiotia is the community of bacteria present in milk.
- Technological advances have allowed researchers to identify DNA from many types of bacteria in milk.
- Milk microbiota research is still in the early stages and the methodology can be improved.
- The origin of bacterial DNA in milk is unknown, but several sources, such as bedding, the rumen, and the skin, have been suggested.
- Not enough is known about the milk microbiota to base treatment decisions on microbiota results.

INTRODUCTION

Mastitis is inflammation of the mammary gland detected by increased somatic cell count (SCC) or visible abnormalities in milk and is the most common bacterial disease of adult dairy cattle.[1] Although numerous bacteria can cause mastitis, historically, most mastitis was caused by *Streptococcus* spp or *Staphylococcus* spp. Mastitis control is improved when programs are targeted at the most prevalent agents. To ensure accurate diagnosis, standardized culturing methods for milk samples have been developed.[2,3] Veterinarians and producers use these results to choose when to use antimicrobial therapy and to ensure the best possible economic outcomes.[4,5] In recent years, scientific advances have led to development of culture-independent technologies that allow for the detection of bacterial DNA in culture-negative milk samples. Some researchers hope sequencing technology will allow for the detection of pathogenic bacteria that were not previously known to cause mastitis. Additionally,

The author has nothing to disclose.
[a] Department of Dairy Science, University of Wisconsin-Madison, 1675 Observatory Drive, Madison, WI 53706, USA; [b] Department of Medical Microbiology and Immunology, University of Wisconsin-Madison, 1550 Linden Drive, Madison, WI 53706, USA; [c] Department of Bacteriology, University of Wisconsin-Madison, 1550 Linden Drive, Madison, WI 53706, USA; [d] Department of Animal Sciences, Michigan State University, 484 S Shaw Lane, E. Lansing, MI 48824, USA
* Corresponding author.
E-mail address: plruegg@msu.edu

some researchers believe the detection of DNA from many types of bacteria indicates mastitis may be a multiagent disease, as opposed to the conventional concept that mastitis is generally caused by a single pathogen.[6,7] This article describes why the milk microbiota has become a topic of interest and how the milk microbiota is analyzed, with the goal of helping veterinarians understand limitations and advantages of microbiota research.

TERMINOLOGY

Much of the terminology used in modern microbiological research may be unfamiliar to most practicing veterinarians. Important terms and their definitions include the following:

Microbiota: communities of microbes within a system.[8] This review addresses bacterial communities, but viruses, archaea, and fungi also contribute to the microbiota.

Microbiome: genomes of the organisms of the microbiota.[8]

Sterile: free of viable microorganisms.

Operational taxonomic unit (OTU): a proxy for "species" used to classify bacteria. Depending on the method used, classification of organisms may come at any taxonomic level from kingdom to species. OTU is used when referring to the various classification levels.[9]

Richness: this term is one of the most common ways that OTUs are described and refers to a calculated metric that accounts for the number of OTUs in a sample.[10] Richness is a basic descriptor of the microbiota.

Diversity: a calculated metric that accounts for the number and evenness of OTUs in a sample.[10,11] Diversity, like richness, is a commonly used basic descriptor of the microbiota.

Polymerase chain reaction (PCR): a laboratory method in which DNA is approximately doubled in each cycling step.

Primer: a short strand of DNA that is complementary to the gene being amplified in PCR. The primer provides a starting point from which the polymerase can add more nucleotides.

Polymerase: the enzyme that adds new nucleotides to DNA during PCR.

Sequencing: determining the order of nucleotides in a strand of DNA.

HISTORICAL UNDERSTANDING OF THE MILK MICROBIOTA

When scientists and veterinarians initially began culturing dairy cow milk, *Streptococcus agalactiae* and *Staphylococcus aureus* were the most common agents of mastitis and these organisms were frequently recovered from milk samples. As milking hygiene improved and the etiologies shifted toward environmental pathogens, the proportion of milk samples from which no bacteria grew in culture increased.[3,12] Reasons for increased proportion of culture-negative milk samples vary but include the decline in prevalence of easily cultured *S agalactiae*. As the proportion of infected quarters declined, researchers concluded culture-negative milk collected from quarters with low SCC was sterile and did not contain a normal flora.[13] Recently, researchers have begun to question the concept of milk sterility, because initial studies using culture-independent sequencing technologies have revealed a wide variety of bacterial DNA in milk samples collected from healthy and inflamed quarters.[7,14–16] However, although bacterial DNA are recovered from many culture-negative milk samples, the origin of the DNA is unknown. Possible sources of the DNA found in milk include bacteria introduced from the cow's skin or environment during sample collection, bacteria or bacterial DNA trapped within the keratin of the teat canal, bacteria or bacterial DNA within leukocytes in milk, and bacteria found in the milk within the mammary gland.[17] The source of bacterial DNA in samples is important because if the bacterial DNA did not come from the milk within the mammary gland, the bacteria may not have been related to mammary health outcomes. To date, there are few published papers describing the milk microbiota and the understanding of this topic will likely improve as methods for detection and analysis of bacteria in milk continue to evolve.

HOW THE MILK MICROBIOTA IS DETERMINED
Sample Collection

To understand how to interpret the milk microbiota, one must understand how the microbiota is detected. The first step of microbiota analysis is sample collection (**Fig. 1**). The National Mastitis Council recommends using an iodine pre-dip as part of the teat-sanitizing process before milk sample collection. After the sanitizing iodine is removed, teats are scrubbed with isopropanol.[2] Even with two sanitizing steps, collecting clean milk samples in a milking parlor or barn is difficult. Sample collection is the first of many opportunities to introduce contaminant DNA into microbiota samples, and therefore must be performed carefully.[18] Because bacterial DNA used in these methods is extracted from milk and amplified with PCR before analysis, contamination with even a few colonies can give misleading results. Minimizing the opportunity for contamination during collection, sample handling, and in the laboratory is essential when using molecular techniques. Contaminant DNA introduced into samples may drown out noncontaminant DNA, especially in samples with a sparse bacterial population, such as milk.[19]

Milk samples should be cultured before microbiota analysis to identify viable bacteria and verify that samples are not contaminated. Contamination rates in culture-based mastitis studies range from approximately 5%[20,21] to more than 15%.[22,23] Some milk microbiota researchers have not cultured milk samples,[24–26] which makes microbiota analysis results difficult to interpret because an unknown proportion of samples either contained viable bacteria or were likely contaminated (**Table 1**). Rainard[17] mentioned that microbiota analysis cannot determine the source of bacterial DNA sequences found in milk and recommended collecting milk directly from the mammary gland cistern to verify that bacterial DNA is found in the cisternal milk and microbiota studies are not merely reporting on bacterial DNA introduced into milk from outside the mammary gland. Collection of milk samples from the gland cistern using a needle and vacuum tube has been used to evaluate the use of PCR for mastitis diagnosis.[27] Samples collected directly from the gland cistern had less bacterial DNA and required more PCR cycles to detect bacterial DNA as compared with samples collected manually;

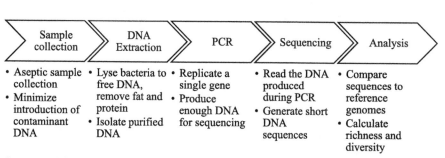

Fig. 1. Workflow for microbiota analysis.

Table 1
Comparison of methods for detecting bacteria in milk

	Culturing	PCR Kit	Microbiota Analysis
Scope of detection	Live bacteria that are culturable in the conditions used	Live or dead known mastitis pathogens with primers included in the kit	Any bacteria with a published genome
Availability	Veterinary diagnostic laboratories, on-farm culturing	Veterinary diagnostic laboratories	Research laboratories
Results are used to guide treatment decisions or management strategies	Yes	Yes	No

manually collected samples also had fewer bacterial species detected.[27] However, this technique is invasive (**Fig. 2**), requires sedation, and is not practical for clinical work. Recent research using this technique demonstrated that bacterial DNA is present in samples collected without being exposed the teat canal, teat skin, or environment, even in milk collected from healthy cows with a low SCC.[16]

DNA Extraction, Polymerase Chain Reaction, and Sequencing

After samples are collected, DNA must be extracted so that the purified DNA can then be amplified to be sufficient for sequencing (see **Fig. 1**). Many DNA extraction kits are commercially available, and some are designed for specific types of samples, such as feces or soil. The selection of an extraction method for milk samples is an important step in the laboratory process because milk contains far less bacterial DNA than rumen or fecal samples.[28] Milk microbiota researchers have not reached a consensus on extraction methods, which has led to the use of a wide variety of DNA extraction methods. Some groups have used kits developed for DNA extraction from soil samples,[26] whereas others have used kits intended for bodily fluid DNA extraction.[14,29] Different kits do not extract DNA equally from all types of bacteria, which may bias results in favor of certain types of bacteria and distort results.[30] This issue has been recognized in earlier research and The Human Microbiome Project has established

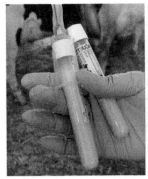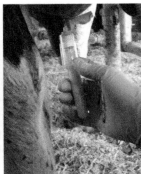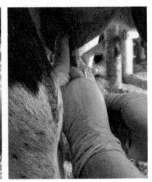

Fig. 2. Cisternal collection of milk samples using a needle and vacuum tube with no additive.

standardized laboratory protocols for working with DNA in microbiota analysis,[31] but milk microbiota analysis has no such standardized protocols. Thus, veterinarians should be cautious when comparing results among different laboratories and research groups.

The next step after extraction of DNA is amplification of that DNA using PCR (see **Fig. 1**). Many veterinarians are familiar with use of PCR as a tool for diagnosis of mastitis pathogens.[32–34] Unlike PCR kits used for identification of common mastitis-causing bacteria, the PCR performed for microbiota analysis does not contain primers targeted toward specific pathogens (see **Table 1**). Instead, microbiota PCR uses universal primers that result in amplification of DNA from any bacteria. Usually, the 16S bacterial small ribosomal subunit gene is selected for PCR amplification because this highly conserved gene is universal among bacteria, ensuring that all bacteria present in the initial sample have DNA amplification. The gene also has variable regions, ensuring that the amplified portions of DNA are useful for discriminating among bacteria when the genes are compared with publicly available genome databases. However, this process does not always have consistent results and differing information may result based on how the amplification process is performed. The number of PCR cycles used for amplification is an important laboratory decision that has varied among studies. Each PCR cycle approximately doubles the amount of DNA, and the cycle number required for milk samples contrasts with bacteria-dense environments, such as rumen contents or feces, which contain enough bacteria that 25 cycles is sufficient for successful PCR amplification.[28] Milk microbiota researchers have used 30, 35, or 40 PCR cycles. Indeed, the bacterial load is so low in healthy milk that some groups have had to perform an extra PCR step before ribosomal-targeted PCR[14] or have reported failed PCR amplification indicating that little bacterial DNA could be extracted from the milk samples.[16,26] After the chosen gene is amplified with PCR, the PCR products are sequenced to identify the source bacteria (see **Fig. 1**). Sequencing methods have improved, and early researchers used methods that are now outdated, limiting comparability of older and newer studies. Initial researchers used pyrosequencing[6,7,14,15,29] and the current standard is Illumina sequencing.[16,25,26] Pyrosequencing provided OTU at a higher resolution (eg, genus rather than family)[35] but was significantly more expensive than Illumina sequencing[36] and is no longer supported by the company that owns the technology.[37]

Identification is made when a DNA sequence matches a reference genome (see **Fig. 1**).[38] The alignment to the reference database can come at any taxonomic level. Generally, as the length and quality of a DNA sequence increases, the alignment comes at a deeper taxonomic level (eg, genus rather than phylum). Sequence results are described in terms of the number of OTU, rather than species, because the results contain many types of bacteria identified at various taxonomic levels from kingdom to species. For example, some sequences may be assigned to an OTU at the genus level *Staphylococcus*. Many species of *Staphylococcus* are important mastitis pathogens but knowing whether an animal is infected with *S aureus* or a non-*aureus Staphylococcus* species is vital for making a treatment decision.[39] Non-*aureus Staphylococcus* species are more likely to be eliminated by antimicrobial therapy, whereas *S aureus* is difficult to treat and may indicate milking management deficiencies.[39] The best identification provided by Illumina sequencing usually comes at the genus level, rather than the species level, which limits the applicability of results.

Two of the most common descriptors used in microbiota analysis are richness and diversity. "Richness" accounts for the number of OTU in a sample; "diversity" accounts for the number and evenness of OTU (**Fig. 3**). Samples with DNA sequences from more OTU have greater richness, and samples that are not dominated by few OTU have greater diversity (see **Fig. 3**). There are numerous ways to calculate richness and diversity, each of which account for low-frequency sequences in different

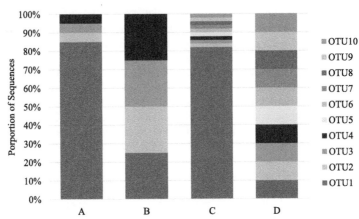

Fig. 3. Example of richness and diversity metrics. Richness is low in A and B, with only four OTUs present. Richness is greater in C and D, with 10 OTUs present. Diversity, which accounts for evenness and number of OTUs, is greater in B than in A, and greater in D than in B.

ways.[10,11] The important point to remember when reading about richness and diversity is that greater richness and diversity are generally associated with better health outcomes in systems with a well-characterized dense microbiota, such as the gut or skin.[40,41] Although bovine milk from healthy quarters seems to contain far less bacterial DNA than other communities,[28] researchers are hopeful that richness and diversity metrics will in the future be used to predict which animals are at greater risk for developing mastitis or to predict outcomes after occurrence of mastitis. At this point, most studies have not examined richness and diversity across lactation or in association with cow factors and the environment (**Table 2**), so it is not yet known whether richness and diversity will be more informative than well-known risk factors, such as parity or stage of lactation, for predicting mastitis risk.

MILK MICROBIOTA RESEARCH

The first study of the bovine milk microbiota as described by pyrosequencing was published in 2012.[6] The researchers examined the milk microbiota of subclinically infected Kankrej, Gir, or crossbred cattle with culture-positive milk. *Pseudomonas* spp and *Shigella* spp were among the OTUs detected via sequencing, along with the *S aureus* and *Escherichia coli* that were found with sequencing and culturing. The results of this study illustrated that many OTUs could be detected in milk, even beyond those that were cultured, but the study had a different sample population of Bos indicus cattle than the Bos taurus cattle found on most North American dairies[6] and interpretation of results of this study is limited because of inadequate description of the cows and housing conditions.

The milk microbiota of North American dairy cows was first described in 2012.[7] Milk samples that had been collected by dairy producers from cows with subclinical or clinical mastitis and submitted to a mastitis diagnostic laboratory were analyzed along with a group of milk samples from healthy cows that had been collected by the researchers.[7] The sample collection methods used by producers are unknown and the cows' housing are not described. Differences in sample collection methods among producers is an important issue to consider when interpreting results, especially because researchers collecting samples specifically for microbiota analysis are likely to be more careful in using aseptic technique. When assessing culture-positive milk

Table 2
Study design and sample populations of dairy cow milk microbiota studies

Authors	Study Design	Number of Milk Samples	Type of Milk Samples	Culturing	Location	Cow Populations
Bhatt et al,[6] 2012	Cross-sectional observational study	120 were collected; the number sequenced is not reported	Quarter-milk	Yes	Gujarat State, India	Kankrej, Gir, and crossbred cows
Oikonomou et al,[7] 2012	Cross-sectional observational study	136 with clinical or subclinical mastitis, 20 healthy	Healthy milk samples were quarter samples; mastitis samples are not described	Yes	Unknown; submitted to a laboratory in New York	Unknown
Kuehn et al,[14] 2013	Cross-sectional observational study	10 with clinical mastitis, 10 nonclinical from the same cows, 2 low SCC quarters from healthy cows	Quarter-milk	Yes	Iowa	Holstein cows
Oikonomou et al,[15] 2014	Cross-sectional observational study	177	Quarter-milk	Yes	New York	Unknown
Young et al,[24] 2015	Cross-sectional observational study	12	Either quarter or composite, collected via teat cannula	No	Waikato, New Zealand	Friesian, Jersey, or Friesian × Jersey
Falentin et al,[29] 2016	Cross-sectional retrospective cohort study	31	Quarter-milk with teat swabs	Yes	France	Primiparous Holstein cows
Ganda et al,[25] 2016	Randomized controlled trial	Possibly 640; 8 time points, possibly 80 quarters	Quarter-milk	Mastitis samples only	New York	Holstein cows
Lima et al,[26] 2017	Prospective cohort study	280	Quarter-colostrum	No	New York	Holstein cows
Metzger et al,[16] 2018	Cross-sectional observational study	20 composite, 20 quarter-milk, and 40 cisternal milk	Healthy milk	Yes	Wisconsin	Primiparous Holstein cows

samples, the cultured bacteria were nearly always among the top OTUs found with sequencing.[7] DNA from anaerobic bacteria was detected in mastitis milk samples.[7,15] These anaerobic genera, such as *Fusobacterium* and *Bacteroidetes*, would not be detected with standard aerobic culture conditions, even if the DNA originated from bacteria that were viable within the mammary gland.[2] Anaerobic bacteria are common members of the rumen microbiota, and the presence of DNA from rumen microbes has been used to suggest that a pathway exists that transports gut microbes to the mammary gland.[42] However, at this point, this hypothesis has not been verified.

Four "core" OTUs were found in healthy milk in two studies.[7,15] The researchers referred to the OTUs as "core" members of the microbiota because the OTUs were found in all samples of culture-negative, low-SCC milk. The four OTUs were *Faecalibacterium* spp, *Lachnospiraceae* spp, *Propionibacterium* spp, and *Aeribacillus* spp.[7,15] If confirmed in other studies, a core healthy microbiota would be a target for predicting which cows will develop mastitis. However, the same "core" genera have not been reported in other studies and overall, there is little consistency in OTUs reported by different groups.[14,16,29] A different study reported healthy milk contained *Pseudomonas* spp and *Ralstonia* spp.[14] However, *Pseudomonas* spp are unlikely to be a major contributor to the healthy milk microbiota because *Pseudomonas* spp are mastitis pathogens that can cause rapid increases in SCC and development of clinical mastitis.[43] Potential sources of *Pseudomonas* DNA in milk samples include farm water sources and laboratory reagent contamination. *Pseudomonas* is one of several OTUs that have been found as contaminants in laboratory reagents. Polymerases used as part of the PCR step may contain tiny amounts of bacterial DNA that are duplicated when many cycles are required to amplify the DNA for microbiota analysis.[16,19,24] To avoid polymerase contamination, negative control subjects should be sequenced along with milk samples so that contaminant DNA from negative control subjects are removed from milk sample results.[16,19,24] If contaminant sequences are not removed, contaminant OTUs may dominate the results and cause inaccurate calculations of richness and diversity. In a recent study, after removal of contaminant sequences from *Pseudomonas* and several other OTUs, *Enhydrobacter*, *Prevotella*, and *Janthinobacterium* were among the major OTUs found in low-SCC, culture-negative milk.[16] These OTUs have not been reported in other studies and variation among studies of the healthy milk microbiota may be caused by methodologic differences. However, farm effects, bedding effects, and geography must all be considered in addition to different laboratory methods, because bedding type is associated with the overall bacterial community composition of milk samples collected from healthy cows.[16] Canonical discriminant analysis combines the overall number of sequences from each OTU into two variables; the overall community composition differs by bedding type, with recycled and new sand having similar populations (**Fig. 4**).[16] Researchers should describe the environment and housing of cows used in studies of the milk microbiota to avoid misleading conclusions about origin.

The milk microbiota exhibits a similar trend in community composition to other systems,[40,41] in that the microbiota of healthy milk generally has greater richness and diversity than the microbiota of milk from glands with mastitis,[15,25] even in different mammary glands within the same cow.[14] Healthier microbial communities are not dominated by a few OTUs. A study of the teat microbiota, in which researchers collected foremilk samples and swabs of the teat canal, revealed that diversity was also greater in samples from healthy quarters that had never experienced clinical mastitis as compared with quarters that had experienced a case of clinical mastitis at any point in the past.[29] These studies cannot determine whether microbiota changes precede the development of mastitis, or whether the influx of leukocytes into the mammary gland precedes the changes in the microbiota. Therefore, these

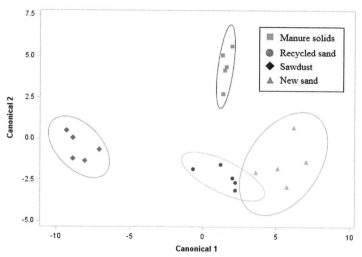

Fig. 4. Canonical discriminant analysis of the top 15 OTUs of milk samples collected using cisternal puncture (n = 20) by bedding type in the cow's pen with 68% prediction ellipses around each group. Milk samples were collected with needle and vacuum tube from cows housed within a single barn in four pens, each with one bedding type: manure solids (n = 5), recycled sand (n = 5), sawdust (n = 5), and new sand (n = 5). (*From* Metzger SA, Hernandez LL, Skarlupka JH, et al. Influence of sampling technique and bedding type on the milk microbiota: results of a pilot study. J Dairy Sci 2018;101:6346–56; with permission.)

data cannot yet be used to predict which animals will develop mastitis or to produce prognoses.

MILK MICROBIOTA ORIGINS

Sequencing technology can tell whether bacterial DNA is present in milk samples but not whether the DNA came from viable bacteria. The prevalence of rumen-associated bacteria, such as *Clostridium* spp or *Ruminococcus* spp, has been used to suggest a pathway between the rumen and the mammary gland. *Lactobacillus fermentum* or *Lactobacillus salivarius* have been cultured from human milk after oral administration of these bacterial species to treat lactational mastitis.[44] A similar gut-mammary pathway has been suggested in cattle[24,42] but has not yet been demonstrated, because the mere presence of bacterial DNA in both the feces and milk does not confirm that the bacterial DNA is entering the mammary gland from the gut. Gut bacteria DNA could also enter the mammary gland through the teat canal from the dairy cow's environment. The udder may be exposed to fecal bacteria when the cow is lying down, and SCC[45] and teat skin bacterial counts[46] are greater in cows with dirtier legs and udders. Skin-associated bacteria could also enter the mammary gland via the teat canal. Milk samples collected directly from the gland cistern (bypassing the teat end) did not contain DNA from many common skin-associated bacteria,[16] such as *Propionibacterium* spp, *Corynebacterium* spp, or *Staphylococcus* spp.[47,48] This lack of skin-associated bacteria in cisternal milk suggests that some of the skin-associated sequences reported in the milk microbiota may be introduced into the milk from the skin during the sample collection process.[16,17,27] At this point, there are insufficient data available to draw conclusions about the presence or purpose of a bovine milk microbiota. Variation in laboratory and sampling methods precludes comparison of results among studies and limits the ability to determine potential clinical applications.

APPLICATIONS OF MILK MICROBIOTA RESEARCH

Milk microbiota research is still in the early stages. One obvious goal for milk micro-biota research is to perform microbiota transplants similar to rumen transplantation that has been performed for hundreds of years[49] or the human fecal transplants that are a more recent development for treatment of *Clostridium difficile* infections.[50] Transplantation of the bovine milk microbiome has not been attempted on the same scale as with the rumen microbiome. Milk microbiota transplantations would be difficult because of the physiology of the mammary gland. Unlike the gut, the mammary gland does not have a mucosal layer to protect the epithelium against bacteria and deliberately introducing bacteria into the gland generally causes mastitis.

SUMMARY

The milk microbiota is poorly understood and there is considerable variation in the methods and results of studies conducted to date. Much more research is required before veterinary practitioners will be able to use these technologies for either diag-nostic or clinical applications. Published milk microbiota research using sequencing technologies that should be a stepping stone to further investigations into the viability and importance of the bacteria detected in the milk and the milk microbiota is not yet sufficiently understood for clinical applications.

REFERENCES

1. USDA, Animal and Plant Health Inspection Service. Reference of dairy cattle health and management practices in the United States, 2007. USDA-APHIS-VS, CEAH. Fort Collins, CO #N480.1007.
2. National Mastitis Council. Laboratory handbook on bovine mastitis. New Prague (MN): National Mastitis Council; 2017.
3. Ruegg PL. A 100-year review: mastitis detection, management, and prevention. J Dairy Sci 2017;100(12):10381–97.
4. Pinzón-Sánchez C, Cabrera VE, Ruegg PL. Decision tree analysis of treatment strategies for mild and moderate cases of clinical mastitis occurring in early lacta-tion. J Dairy Sci 2011;94(4):1873–92.
5. Lago A, Godden SM, Bey R, et al. The selective treatment of clinical mastitis based on on-farm culture results: I. Effects on antibiotic use, milk withholding time, and short-term clinical and bacteriological outcomes. J Dairy Sci 2011; 94(4):4441–56.
6. Bhatt VD, Ahir VB, Koringa PG, et al. Milk microbiome signatures of subclinical mastitis-affected cattle analysed by shotgun sequencing. J Appl Microbiol 2012;112(4):639–50.
7. Oikonomou G, Machado VS, Santisteban C, et al. Microbial diversity of bovine mastitic milk as described by pyrosequencing of metagenomics 16s rDNA. PLoS One 2012;7(10):e47671.
8. Turnbaugh PJ, Ley RE, Hamady M, et al. The human microbiome project. Nature 2007;449(7164):804–10.
9. Blaxter M, Mann J, Chapman T, et al. Defining operational taxonomic units using DNA barcode data. Philos Trans R Soc Lond B Biol Sci 2005;360(1462):1935–43.
10. Kindt R, Coe R. Tree diversity analysis: a manual and software for common sta-tistical methods for ecological and biodiversity studies. Nairobi (Kenya): World Agroforestry Centre (ICRAF); 2005.

11. Colwell K. Biodiversity: concepts, patterns, and measurement. The Princeton guide to ecology. Princeton (NJ): Princeton University Press; 2009. p. 257–63.
12. Neave FK, Dodd FH, Kingwill RG, et al. Control of mastitis in the dairy herd by hygiene and management. J Dairy Sci 1969;52(5):696–707.
13. Dodd FH, Neave FK, Kingwill RG. Control of udder infection by management. J Dairy Sci 1964;47(10):1109–14.
14. Kuehn JS, Gorden PJ, Munro D, et al. Bacterial community profiling of milk samples as a means to understand culture-negative bovine clinical mastitis. PLoS One 2013;8(4):e61959.
15. Oikonomou G, Bicalho ML, Meira E, et al. Microbiota of cow's milk: distinguishing healthy, sub-clinically, and clinically diseased quarters. PLoS One 2014;9(1):e85904.
16. Metzger SA, Hernandez LL, Skarlupka JH, et al. Influence of sampling technique and bedding type on the milk microbiota: results of a pilot study. J Dairy Sci 2018; 101:1–11.
17. Rainard P. Mammary microbiota of dairy ruminants: fact or fiction? Vet Res 2017; 48(1):25.
18. Salter SJ, Cox MJ, Turek EM, et al. Reagent and laboratory contamination can critically impact sequence-based microbiome analyses. BMC Biol 2014;12:87.
19. Jervis-Bardy J, Leong LEX, Marri S, et al. Deriving accurate microbiota profiles from human samples with low bacterial content through post-sequencing processing of Illumina MiSeq data. Microbiome 2015;3:19.
20. Koivula M, Pitkälä A, Pyörälä S, et al. Distribution of bacteria and seasonal and regional effects in a new database for mastitis pathogens in Finland. Acta Agr Scand Sec A - Animal Science 2007;57(2):89–96.
21. Oliveira L, Ruegg PL. Treatments of clinical mastitis occurring in cows on 51 large dairy herds in Wisconsin. J Dairy Sci 2014;97(9):5426–36.
22. Makovec JA, Ruegg PL. Results of milk samples submitted for microbiological examination in Wisconsin from 1194 to 2001. J Dairy Sci 2003;86(11):3466–72.
23. Persson Y, Nyman A-K, Grönlund-Andersson U. Etiology and antimicrobial susceptibility of udder pathogens from cases of subclinical mastitis in dairy cows in Sweden. Acta Vet Scand 2011;53(1):36.
24. Young W, Hine BC, Wallace OAM, et al. Transfer of intestinal bacterial components to mammary secretions in the cow. PeerJ 2015;3:e888.
25. Ganda EK, Bisinotto RF, Lima SF, et al. Longitudinal metagenomic profiling of bovine milk to assess the impact of intramammary treatment using a third-generation cephalosporin. Sci Rep 2016;6:37565.
26. Lima SF, Teixeira AGV, Lima FS, et al. The bovine colostrum microbiome and its association with clinical mastitis. J Dairy Sci 2017;100(4):3031–42.
27. Hiitiö H, Simojoki H, Kalmus P, et al. The effect of sampling technique on PCR-based bacteriological results of bovine milk samples. J Dairy Sci 2016;99(8): 6532–41.
28. Dill-McFarland KA, Breaker JD, Suen G. Microbial succession in the gastrointestinal tract of dairy cows from 2 weeks to first lactation. Sci Rep 2017;7:40864.
29. Falentin H, Rault L, Nicolas S, et al. Bovine teat microbiome analysis revealed reduced alpha diversity and significant changes in taxonomic profiles in quarters with a history of mastitis. Front Microbiol 2016;7:480.
30. Quigley L, O'Sullivan O, Beresford TP, et al. A comparison of methods used to extract bacterial DNA from raw milk and raw milk cheese. J Appl Microbiol 2012;113(1):96–105.
31. McInnes P, Cutting M. Manual of procedures for human microbiome project, core microbiome sampling, protocol A, HMP protocol # 07-001. 2010.

32. Taponen S, Salmikivi L, Simojoki H, et al. Real-time polymerase chain reaction-based identification of bacteria in milk samples from bovine clinical mastitis with no growth in conventional culturing. J Dairy Sci 2009;92(6):2610–7.

33. Koskinen MT, Wellenberg GJ, Sampimon OC, et al. Field comparison of real-time polymerase chain reaction and bacterial culture for identification of bovine mastitis bacteria. J Dairy Sci 2010;93(12):5707–15.

34. Viora L, Graham EM, Mellor DJ, et al. Evaluation of a culture-based pathogen identification kit for bacterial causes of bovine mastitis. Vet Rec 2014;175(4):89.

35. Claesson MJ, Wang Q, O'Sullivan O, et al. Comparison of two next-generation sequencing technologies for resolving highly complex microbiota composition using tandem variable 16S rRNA gene regions. Nucleic Acids Res 2010;38(22):e200.

36. Shendure J, Ji H. Next-generation DNA sequencing. Nat Biotechnol 2008;26(10):1135–45.

37. Genomeweb. Roche shutting down 454 sequencing business. Available at: https://www.genomeweb.com/sequencing/roche-shutting-down-454-sequencing-business#.WwSULUgvzIV. Accessed May 22, 2018.

38. DeSantis TZ, Hugenholt P, Larsen N, et al. Greengenes, a chimera-checked 16S rRNA gene database and workbench compatible with ARB. Appl Environ Microbiol 2006;72(7):5069–72.

39. Taponen S, Pyörälä S. Coagulase-negative staphylococci as cause of bovine mastitis: not so different from *Staphylococcus aureus*? Vet Microbiol 2009;134(1–2):29–36.

40. Kong HH, Oh J, Deming C, et al. Temporal shifts in the skin microbiome associated with disease flares and treatment in children with atopic dermatitis. Genome Res 2012;22(5):850–9.

41. Cho I, Blaser MJ. The human microbiome: at the interface of health and disease. Nat Rev Genet 2012;13(4):260–70.

42. Addis MF, Tanca A, Uzzau S, et al. The bovine milk microbiota: insights and perspectives from -omics studies. Mol Biosyst 2016;12:2359–72.

43. Bannerman DD, Chockalingam A, Paape MJ, et al. The bovine innate immune response during experimentally-induced *Pseudomonas aeruginosa* mastitis. Vet Immunol Immunopathol 2005;107(3–4):201–15.

44. Arroyo R, Martin RV, Maldonado A, et al. Treatment of infectious mastitis during lactation: antibiotics versus oral administration of lactobacilli isolated from breast milk. Clin Infect Dis 2010;50(12):1551–8.

45. Schreiner DA, Ruegg PL. Relationship between udder and leg hygiene scores and subclinical mastitis. J Dairy Sci 2003;86(11):3460–5.

46. Guarín JF, Baumberger C, Ruegg PL. Anatomical characteristics of teats and pre-milking bacterial counts of teat skin swabs of primiparous cows exposed to different types of bedding. J Dairy Sci 2017;100(2):1436–44.

47. Braem GS, De Vliegher S, Verbist B, et al. Culture-independent exploration of the teat apex microbiota of dairy cows reveals a wide bacterial species diversity. Vet Microbiol 2012;157(3–4):383–90.

48. Braem G, De Vliegher S, Verbist B, et al. Unraveling the microbiota of teat apices of clinically healthy lactating dairy cows, with special emphasis on coagulase-negative staphylococci. J Dairy Sci 2013;96(3):1499–510.

49. Brag S, Hansen HJ. Treatment of ruminal indigestion according to popular belief in Sweden. Rev Sci Tech 1994;13(2):529–35.

50. Gough E, Shaikh H, Manges AR. Systematic review of intestinal microbiota transplantation (fecal bacteriotherapy) for recurrent *Clostridium difficile* infection. Clin Infect Dis 2011;53(10):994–1002.

Mastitis Control in Automatic Milking Systems

John F. Penry, BVSc, MVS, PhD

KEYWORDS

- Mastitis • Automatic milking system • Detection systems • Sensor • Cow

KEY POINTS

- Milking, and initial mastitis detection in an Automatic milking system is automated and does not involve human input. Milking is typically quarter based.
- There are mastitis control risk factors common to both conventional and automatic milking systems: environmental contamination, teat congestion and teat hyperkeratosis risk.
- Certain mastitis control risk factors will differ between conventional and automatic milking systems: pre-milking preparation, impact formation, and overmilking risk.
- Mastitis sensor system performance should include a robust description of test sensitivity, success rate and false alert rate along with the gold standard used.
- The most common sensor systems used incorporate a measurement of electrical conductivity in isolation, or with other data, to determine an alert.

Automatic milking systems (AMSs), sometimes referred to as robotic milking systems, were first commercially introduced in the Netherlands in 1992. Since that time, the number of AMS units deployed on farms worldwide has grown to around 38,000,[1] with most AMSs being located in western Europe and North America. A single AMS unit typically services between 50 and 70 animals either as a single unit available to 1 group of cows or multiple units in 1 barn servicing a larger group. Optimal efficiency for a unit is when the AMS is occupied for milking approximately 80% of each 24-hour period.[2] AMSs are typically associated with free-stall housing systems, although they are also found in countries with predominantly pasture-based dairying where animals are not routinely housed.

The development and uptake of AMS has primarily been driven by 3 factors: first, advances in robotic technology and its application to biological systems; second, the desire to reduce repetitive manual tasks on dairy farms; and third, the increasing difficulties seen in many dairying countries around supply and employment of a suitable farm workforce.

Irrespective of whether a cow is milked using an AMS or conventional milking, the same rules about suitability of milk for human consumption apply. In the European Union (EU), EU Directive EC/853/2004 (2004) states that the milker must visually inspect milk from each cow before milking and withhold delivery into the bulk tank if

Cognosco-Anexa FVC, 25 Moorhouse Street, Morrinsville 3340, New Zealand
E-mail address: jpenry@anexafvc.co.nz

Vet Clin Food Anim 34 (2018) 439–456
https://doi.org/10.1016/j.cvfa.2018.06.004
0749-0720/18/© 2018 Elsevier Inc. All rights reserved.

abnormalities indicating intramammary infection (IMI) or color change can be seen.[3] Detection and discarding of milk with visual signs of abnormality is also mandated through the US Food and Drug Administration (FDA) Grade A Pasteurized Milk Ordinance[4] with similar requirements for withholding of abnormal milk from the bulk tank operating in other dairying countries.

Mastitis control on farms using AMSs can be thought of as similar to farms using conventional milking in that many of the primary control points preventing new IMI are the same. The 2 milk harvesting systems differ, though, in detection of clinical mastitis (CM).

DIFFERENCES IN MILK HARVESTING BETWEEN CONVENTIONAL MILKING AND AUTOMATIC MILKING SYSTEMS

There are distinct, and important, differences between milk harvesting practices in AMSs compared with conventional milking:

- Farm staff are not routinely involved in milking operations in AMSs
- Cows determine their own milking frequency, or milking interval (MI) with the proviso that a typical AMS operation incorporates milking permission, which depends on anticipated milk yield (MY), MI, or a combination of the two
- Teat premilking preparation is fully automated and highly consistent, in terms of routine application, in AMSs
- Detection of abnormal milk and diversion from the bulk tank is automated in AMSs and relies on sensor systems and related information support processes
- Milk harvesting is at the quarter level in AMSs with milk not passing through a cluster immediately under the 4 teat cups
- Teat-cup detachment is controlled at the quarter level
- AMSs are typically not designed for easy, or safe, farm staff access to the teat and udder during routine operation, making milk collection for culture difficult

Milk Quality Trends Seen When Changing from Conventional Milking to Automatic Milking Systems

Numerous studies have examined milk quality and udder health trends, comparing conventional milking with AMS or following farms shifting from conventional milking to AMS. In summary, the trend is for deterioration of udder health metrics such as CM prevalence and proportion of the herd with an increased individual cow somatic cell count (ICSCC) in AMSs.[5] In a 69-farm Danish study, the bulk tank somatic cell count (BTSCC) increased during a period of adaptation after introduction of AMS with the proportion of cows with an increased ICSCC persisting for the first year.[6] A larger study, also conducted in Denmark, described an overall increase in ICSCC 4 years after the introduction of AMSs on 478 farms.[7] Eighty-eight Finnish herds that changed to AMS were compared with around 200 conventional milking herds and showed a higher average ICSCC in the first year after AMS integration.[8] An increase in the use of antibiotics for IMI treatment was described by Bennedsgaard and colleagues[9] on 20 farms and this, in part, may have been driven by responses to the mastitis alert system after AMS introduction. Of the studies reviewed by Hovinen and Pyorala,[5] the increase in somatic cell count (SCC) (weighted average day ICSCC or BTSCC) after conversion to AMS ranged between 8000 and 44,000 cells/mL. Interpretation of studies examining mastitis control after the switch from conventional milking to AMS have to be undertaken carefully because the changes made often involve more than just the milking system and can include housing and laneway alterations.[5]

MASTITIS CONTROL FACTORS COMMON TO CONVENTIONAL MILKING AND AUTOMATIC MILKING SYSTEMS

Reducing the new IMI rate, when described in first principles, is about decreasing the number of mastitis-causing bacteria around the teat and maintaining optimal teat-end and teat-tissue health. In this regard, there are numerous mastitis control points that are exactly the same, irrespective of the milking system in use.

Controlling Environmental Contamination of the Teats and Udder

Limiting the degree of environmental contamination around teat tissue and the udder has been the focus of research for many years. An early study by Neave and colleagues[10] found an association between the incidence of IMI and the number of mastitis pathogens around the teat end. Bacterial numbers present in milk increase when teats are not adequately cleaned and dried during premilking preparation.[11] Farms that supplied milk with a lower BTSCC had cleaner cows and housing environments compared with herds with higher BTSCC.[12]

An udder and leg hygiene scoring system described by Schreiner and Ruegg[13] has been incorporated into numerous mastitis control assessment procedures. As detailed in their article, the udder and legs of a representative sample of cows are assessed and scored immediately before milking on a 4-point scale (1 being clean; 4 being very dirty). Significant changes in linear ICSCC were observed in contrast between all scores except between 1 and 2 and between 3 and 4. The prevalence of IMI caused by environmental pathogens was significantly associated with an increasing udder hygiene score. When applied in the field, a target is to have less than 20% of udders score 3 or 4. Application of this scoring system in AMS is more difficult for farm staff, or their advisers, because cows typically can only easily be viewed from the side of the udder immediately before teat-cup attachment. This situation differs from application of this scoring system in a conventional parlor, where, depending on the depth of splash trays above the kicking rail, the udder and legs can be clearly viewed from behind. Hence, interpretation of the hygiene scoring results in AMS has to be done carefully, particularly when benchmarking against other conventional milking facilities because the observation method may not be as complete. Observation in AMS installations may best be achieved around the AMS unit holding area.

Management of free-stall areas, laneways, and holding pens to reduce the amount of environmental contamination is similar in conventional milking facilities and AMS. In both scenarios, efficient removal of effluent, laneway cleanliness, bedding management, free-stall occupation rate, and holding pen cleanliness contribute to minimizing opportunities for legs and udders to become soiled. The premilking holding area in an AMS may be less affected by effluent compared with the holding area around a conventional parlor, but this depends on the area allocated per cow and the automatic milking traffic management system (free, semiguided, or guided).

Teat-End and Teat-Barrel Congestion

There are no differences in the physical forces transmitted, via the liner, to the teat when conventional milking is compared with AMS. Milking vacuum creates a pressure gradient underneath the teat end, thereby unfolding the teat canal and causing milk to flow from the teat sinus into the liner and through the short milk tube. Pulsation, applied via the teat-cup pulsation chamber, is required to provide compression to the teat end, typically at between 55 to 65 cycles/min. This liner compression, in turn, assists the return of blood and lymph from the teat end, where it accumulates because of the forces of vacuum.[14,15] No liner compression is applied to the teat-barrel wall and hence any accumulation of congestion in either the circulatory pathway or the interstitial space in this area of the teat cannot be relieved through the action of the liner.[16]

The formation of teat-end congestion can be caused by an increase in teat-end vacuum.[17,18] It may also be induced where the pulsation b-phase duration is increased where system milking vacuum and liner compression remain constant.[19] Although these changes are short term, conditions that lead to congestion and edema that are allowed to persist over many milkings can cause chronic changes such as ringing at the teat base. Teat congestion has been associated with increases in IMI[20,21] in addition to an increase in ICSCC.[22]

Systems for assessing the degree of teat congestion are described in various national mastitis control programs.[23,24] A sample of cows, representative of the herd, are visually assessed and scored for teat tissue color change, evidence of ringing at the teat base, and petechiae. An aggregated score is then compared with a predetermined threshold level depending on whether the assessment is being done at the cow or quarter level. If there is evidence of teat congestion, beyond the threshold level, further assessment of the milking machine should be undertaken. This further assessment includes teat-end vacuum during the peak milk flow period (milking time test), which should average between the 36 to 42 kPa recommended for gentle milking.[25] Pulsation ratio and rate should be converted into milliseconds for each pulsation phase: the b-phase should not exceed approximately 500 milliseconds to prevent teat canal congestion within a single pulsation cycle[14] and the d-phase should be greater than 150 milliseconds.[26] Liner geometry can also influence the degree of teat-barrel congestion. Ronningen and Postma[27] reported that, for optimal udder health, the vacuum in the mouthpiece chamber should be between 10 and 30 kPa, although results from a more recent study suggest that there may be advantages from having mouthpiece chamber vacuum as low as possible, providing there is no liner slip.[28] It has been proposed that poor fit around the mouthpiece opening or between the teat skin and the liner wall increases mouthpiece chamber vacuum.[27,29]

Applying a visual teat assessment system, after teat-cup detachment, is more difficult in AMS compared with conventional milking parlors. Primarily this is because farm staff, or an adviser, can typically only get access to the cow from 1 side of the udder and a clear view is often hampered by the AMS equipment (robotic arm) and structure at the height of the udder and teats. It is more challenging to get a 90° to 180° view of any individual teat, which may decrease the ease with which teat tissue observations can take place.

In a similar vein, milking time measurements of short milk tube and mouthpiece chamber vacuum with a vacuum recording device (handheld or VaDia) are far more cumbersome in AMSs compared with a conventional cluster because of the action of the robotic arm that places each teat cup from the AMS magazine onto the teat. Although vacuum measurements at various locations around the liner are possible, they often involve placement of the measuring device during an individual cow milking, after teat-cup attachment, when safe physical access to the teat cup is very limited. If teat observations indicate that the level of teat-end or teat-barrel congestion is above the trigger level prompting further investigation, the application of milking time performance tests to assess vacuum during milk flow (short milk tube and mouthpiece chamber) are important to support any recommended changes in milking system vacuum or liner type. At present there are no National Mastitis Council guidelines on milking time performance testing in AMSs, although they are in development.

Teat-End Hyperkeratosis

Teat-end hyperkeratosis (HK) has also been described as teat-end callosity and can be detected on teats, on average, within 8 weeks of calving.[30] It is the result of physical forces applied to the teat end by vacuum and the action of the liner during milking. The widely referenced study by Neijenhuis and colleagues[31] reported a small but significant effect of teat-end HK on the prevalence of CM between the second and fourth months of lactation. Following on from this study, reduction of HK in any herd is seen as a useful control measure in limiting new IMI.

The effects of environment (eg, extreme cold weather) are the overriding ones for the formation of HK,[32] but liner compression is the primary milking machine risk factor.[33] As liner compression increases, so does the risk of HK formation based on survey results with 7 different liners used in US dairies.[32] Increasing system vacuum has the effect of also increasing liner compression for a given liner design. Hence, system vacuum levels designed to achieve fast milk flow rates may have an additive effect on HK risk. Liner compression can be estimated based on a biologically relevant indicator, overpressure,[34] but currently no liner manufacturers report liner overpressure routinely on product description materials.

Mein and colleagues[35] proposed a teat-end HK scoring system that is now in widespread use in milking time evaluation systems. Teat-end HK is scored as N (no ring), S (smooth), R (rough), or VR (very rough) either on an individual quarter basis or using a system in which the worst-scoring teat for a cow becomes the cow's HK score. Irrespective of the scoring system used, HK scores from a representative sample of the herd are then compared with thresholds for the prevalence of R and VR scores. These thresholds, or trigger levels, guide the farm team and their advisers around the need for further investigation into HK risk factors for a herd. The difficulties in thorough teat observation, after teat-cup detachment, identified earlier in this article remain relevant for the assessment of teat-end HK in AMS. If HK scores are beyond threshold levels, the AMS milking configuration should be assessed for both system vacuum and vacuum in the short milk tube during milk flow, if possible, to assess the appropriateness of the vacuum level during milking. If high liner compression is suspected as a contributing cause to HK, a change in liner should be contemplated. However, any change needs to be based on in-the-field knowledge from milking machine technicians, or other advisers, because liner overpressure values are not reported, if measured at all, during initial design and manufacture.

Peak Milk Flow Rate and Mastitis Risk

Over many decades, researchers have examined the association between various milk harvesting indicators, including peak milk flow rate, and mastitis incidence. Peak milk flow rate (kilograms per minute) can be measured either at the udder or quarter level. Dodd and Neave,[36] in the 1950s, found a positive correlation between udder milk flow rate and mastitis incidence in primiparous cows.[36] Supporting this finding, Grindal and Hillerton[37] reported a significant increase in new CM infections when quarter peak milk flow rate was greater than 1.6 kg/min using an experimental challenge model with *Streptococcus agalactiae* and *Streptococcus dysgalactiae*. However, Brown and colleagues[38] found no association between linear somatic cell score (SCS) and udder peak milk flow rate and, similarly, Halley and colleagues[39] did not show a significant correlation between average udder peak milk flow rate and lactation average linear SCS.

Only 2 studies have examined the association between peak milk flow rate and CM risk in AMSs. An Australian study, using a moderate-production pasture-based herd, reported an increased risk of CM associated with high quarter peak milk flow rate in a multivariate analysis.[40] However, in the same study, the univariate analysis found both high and low quarter milk flow rate from days −7 to 0 before the CM episode associated with increased CM risk. No mechanism was proposed by the investigators for this unusual finding. A recent case control study, conducted in a high-production US herd, found no association between CM risk and the peak milk flow rate in the affected quarter.[41]

It is worth reflecting on the potential mechanism underlying any observed association between CM risk and peak milk flow rate. Under constant milking system vacuum and pulsation settings, an increase in peak milk flow rate must result from widening of the teat canal.[26] It could be postulated that an increase in the teat canal cross-sectional area during milking potentially results in delayed refolding and closure of the teat canal epidermis, although this mechanism has never been shown, nor has it been discussed in the literature. Irrespective of conflicting findings in this area, it is reasonable to assume that, in AMSs, peak milk flow rate is only a minor risk factor for CM, if a risk factor at all.

MASTITIS CONTROL FACTORS REFLECTING DIFFERENCES BETWEEN AUTOMATIC MILKING SYSTEMS AND CONVENTIONAL MILKING
Milking Interval and Mastitis Risk

As previously stated, one of the unique features of AMSs compared with conventional milking is that cows largely select their own MI throughout a lactation. Although MI can be altered in conventional milking from $1\times$, $2\times$, $3\times$, or even $4\times$, it is all at the pen/herd level and generally fixed for a defined period in the lactation. In a review article, Stelwagen and colleagues[42] reported that an overall increase in ICSCC, but not in CM, was typically seen when MI was increased as a result of changing from $2\times$ to $1\times$ in conventional milking. When AMS was compared with conventional milking of varying MI, no significant change in ICSCC was observed with either AMS compared with $2\times$ or $3\times$ milking.[43] Fogsgaard and colleagues[44] studied 2 AMS herds and reported an increase in MI in the 4 weeks before CM diagnosis. This finding is in general agreement with an Australian[40] and US study,[41] both conducted in commercial AMS herds, that found an association between increasing MI and CM risk. The US (case control) study reported that, for each hour increase in MI, the odds of CM increased by 6%.[41]

Teat Premilking Preparation and Milk Let-Down

In AMS, teat preparation before teat-cup attachment is automated. Although many AMS manufacturers offer farmers the option of altering the time allocated for preparation of each teat, the basic pattern of teat cleaning and tactile stimulation of teat tissue always follows a set pattern of mechanical actions. It is highly standardized within an AMS unit and the teat cleaning system cannot distinguish between a clean and dirty teat before automated cleaning using whichever system is installed. This system is in contrast with conventional milking, in which milkers have the opportunity to alter premilking preparation tasks in response to visual assessment of teats (and udders) during an individual milking session.

From first principles, the association of poor teat hygiene with increased new IMI should be the same when conventional milking is compared with AMS. Dirty teats before teat-cup attachment were reported as a risk factor for increased average herd ICSCC and the proportion of individual cows with an increased ICSCC in 151 Dutch dairy farms using AMS.[45] Teat cleaning in an AMS may be compromised not simply because it is an automated process but also because the cleaning mechanism may experience technical failures (eg, in teat attachment). AMSs generally use either a brushing mechanism or dedicated cleaning teat cup. In a study using a single AMS, Jago and colleagues[46] reported cleaning technical failures in one-third of cow milkings, which is aligned with a larger 9-AMS-herd study finding a similar level of failure.[47] Abnormal udder and teat structure was associated with cleaning technical failures with brushing mechanisms.[47] The effectiveness of teat cleaning, based on visual assessment, was more variable between study herds than between AMS cleaning mechanisms.[48] When summarized, the literature on teat cleaning in AMS indicates that teat hygiene before milking is the primary determinant of the success of this process as part of the overall AMS milking routine.[5]

Irrespective of the teat cleaning system, oxytocin release caused by tactile teat stimulation, and subsequent milk let-down, is achieved successfully in AMS.[49] This is important in the 60 to 90 seconds before teat-cup attachment in order to commence the movement of alveolar milk down into the udder cistern, thereby avoiding the deleterious effects of teat-cup crawl up the teat after the first minute of milking if let-down has failed. If teat cleaning is switched off in AMS, there is likely to be an increase in overall milking time.[46]

Impacts and New Intramammary Infection

In the late 1960s, an Irish milk harvesting study was the first to show, in a field trial, that unstable vacuum at the cluster was linked to an increase in new IMI.[50] Subsequently, a large body of research conducted by O'Shea and O'Callaghan[51] and O'Shea and colleages[52] described a so-called impact mechanism by which irregular vacuum fluctuations, as the result of a single teat-cup slip, caused a sudden pressure gradient across the cluster bowl and propelled milk droplets against the opened teat canal during milking, with an associated increase in new infection risk.

There is no opportunity for the impact mechanism to be observed in AMSs because the milking process is quarter based with no cluster bowl operating immediately below the liner short milk tubes. In an AMS, each liner has its own long milk line transporting milk to a communal or separate and quarter-based, receival vessel. As such, there is no possibility for large, irregular changes in pressure from one teat cup to an adjacent one. Although high cyclic fluctuations in vacuum still occur during each pulsation cycle as a result of the opening and closing of the liner in all milking machines, these are not important as a mechanism of new infection despite being proposed as a causal factor in the 1970s.[53,54] Note that, in modern conventional milking machines, the impact mechanism is likely to be reduced as a new infection risk factor (or possibly eliminated) because of the increase in average claw volume to greater than 150 mL and short milk tubes with a minimum bore size of 10 to 11 mm.[55]

Overmilking and Mastitis Risk

Individual quarters, within an udder, can be thought of as individuals and largely under the influence of local control mechanisms that are removed from systemic hormonal effects.[56] The quarters have individual milk production and milk flow rate characteristics resulting in milk flow rate patterns that rarely have all quarters completing milking at the same time.[57] As a result, in conventional milking, the degree of overmilking for individual teats can have a major effect on teat tissue health and milking gentleness.[16]

In AMS, normally teat-cup detachment is under quarter-by-quarter control based on a set milk flow rate threshold (set at the quarter level). Quarters often go from the peak milk flow period to a low flow rate within the space of 10 pulsation cycles. Although the delay setting for individual teat-cup removal still needs to be taken into account (after the take-off threshold flow rate has been reached), it is highly unlikely that delirious effects will be seen on teat tissue health in AMS caused by any small degree of overmilking, or teat-cup attachment during low milk flow.

DETECTING MASTITIS IN AUTOMATIC MILKING SYSTEMS
Overview of Sensors and Mastitis Detection Systems

As described earlier, dairy farmers are under regulatory direction (and pressure) to supply milk for human consumption that is free of visual abnormalities, including those commonly associated with CM, such as flakes, clots, and watery milk. In AMS, detection of abnormal milk, which should be diverted from supply into the bulk tank, is largely governed by sensor systems built into the AMS. The sensors, and their accompanying information systems, are the first line of detection before human assessment and potential intervention by farm staff.

A starting point for understanding how these systems operate is the review article by Rutten and colleagues.[58] Sensors in dairy production are attached or nonattached, with all AMS sensor systems being nonattached. Nonattached sensors are then categorized as in-line or on-line sensors, with the difference being that in-line sensors take measures from a continuous flow of biological material from the cow (in this case milk), whereas on-line sensor systems take a sample for analysis. Further to this, the sensor system can be thought of as operating at 4 levels:

1. The sensor incorporates a technique or technology that measures something about the cow
2. Interpretation that summarize changes in sensor measurements and results in information about the health status of the cow
3. Integration of sensor information with other, sensor-derived or nonsensor, information to produce advice
4. Creation of an autonomous decision or farmer-led decision

Most of the literature describing AMS sensor systems deals with levels 1 and 2. The relationship between the sensor, the gold standard (GS) for sensor data interpretation, and any ancillary data from other sources is described by an algorithm.[58]

Sensor systems involved in mastitis detection in AMSs vary in type. From approximately 30 publications, sensor systems have included:

- Electrical conductivity (EC)
- Color
- ICSCC or a proxy measurement for cell count, such as an automated Californian mastitis test (CMT) or rapid mastitis test
- Temperature
- MY
- Hydrolytic enzymes (eg, N-acetyl-beta-D-glucosaminidase) or proteolytic enzymes released as a result of inflammation

In most free-stall AMS installations, cows that are flagged for human assessment following a milking mastitis alert are checked between milkings either in the free stall or a holding pen. In pasture-based AMS installations, assessing animals postalert is more complex, involving segregation of the animal at next AMS presentation or a dedicated fetching from the grazing area. It is common practice for cows undergoing treatment of CM in AMS (following an alert or via another detection method) to be milked using conventional equipment for the period of treatment and, potentially, milk withhold.

Irrespective of sensor system detection performance, farmers and their advisers also need to understand issues around sensor system installation costs, running costs, maintenance requirements, calibration parameters, and equipment robustness.[59] Accurate and timely detection of CM in AMS is important for milk quality, animal welfare, and antimicrobial stewardship.

Assessing and Describing Detection System Performance

A sensor system installed into an AMS can have performance described in the same way as for any other biological test using test sensitivity (SE) and specificity (SP). Both are inherent qualities of the test or, in this case, sensor system being described. SE describes test performance in truly diseased animals, whereas SP describes test performance in truly nondiseased animals. For the purposes of sensor performance description in AMS, a diseased or nondiseased animal should be thought of as a cow that has mastitis at an individual milking.

At this point, it is useful to pause and be careful in what is being described. A cow that is defined as "truly having mastitis" does not provide sufficient clarity for any person trying to understand sensor performance. For example, this description may define a cow infected with a mastitis pathogen (based on milk culture) and classified as a subclinical infection based on visual assessment, or a cow for which the infection status is unknown but she remains classified as a subclinical infection because of ICSCC level, or a cow classified as having CM based on a clearly defined description of the visual signs (and other tests) necessary for this diagnosis. Any review of material describing sensor system performance in an AMS must be specific in describing what is meant if "mastitis case" is used as the GS. An overriding constraint in automated mastitis detection is that there is no continual monitoring of the mastitis infection status of a cow, only discrete observations at set time points normally corresponding with milking.[60]

The International Standards Organization (ISO) describes in ISO/FDIS (Final Draft International Standard) 20966, Annex C (Automatic Milking Installations – Requirements and Testing) methods for assessing abnormal milk that should be withheld from bulk tank supply.[61] This document further describes a minimum standard of 80% SE and 99% SP for detection of abnormal milk.

A diagnostic test can also be described according to positive predictive value, being the proportion of positive test results that are truly diseased. Positive predictive value is not an inherent quality of the test, or sensing system, but is instead influenced by disease prevalence. Both Sherlock and colleagues[60] and Hogeveen and colleagues[62] proposed that positive predictive value should be described as success rate (SR) in AMS sensor systems because it is a more useful descriptor for farm staff.

In a similar vein, these groups of investigators[60,62] have also suggested that sensor system SP is a poor term to use with dairy farmers, in part because of the opportunity for numerical perception to be skewed. For example, an SP of 95% may seem numerically to be high, but a mastitis sensing system with this performance would lead to a frustratingly large number of sensor alerts to be checked that would prove to be disease free. As an alternative, false alert rate (FAR) is proposed as a more intuitive measure of sensor system performance. FAR is defined as the number of false sensor alerts per 1000 cow milkings and is calculated by:

- FAR = 10 × (100% − SP%) per 100 cow milkings[60,62]

The importance of these concepts concerning performance of sensing systems is highlighted in **Tables 1–3**, which use an example adapted from Sherlock and colleagues[60] and consider a 100-cow herd being AMS milked, with an average 12-

Table 1
One-hundred-cow herd, 1000 cow milkings (5 days at average 12-hour milking interval), total clinical mastitis based on gold standard = 25

	CM-Positive Cow Milking	CM-Negative Cow Milking	Total
Test Positive	20	30	50
Test Negative	5	945	950
Total	25	975	1000 cow milkings

Sensitivity = 20/25 = 0.80 (80%). Specificity = 945/975 = 0.969 (96.9%). Positive predictive value (SR) = 20/50 = 0.40 (40%). FAR = 10 × (100% − 96.9%) = 30 per 1000 cow milkings.

Table 2
Same scenario as described in Table 1 but increased false alert rate

	CM-Positive Cow Milking	CM-Negative Cow Milking	Total
Test Positive	20	50	70
Test Negative	5	925	930
Total	25	975	1000 cow milkings

Sensitivity = 20/25 = 0.80 (80%). Specificity = 925/975 = 0.949 (94.9%). Positive predictive value (SR) = 20/70 = 0.29 (29%). FAR = 10 × (100% − 94.9%) = 50 per 1000 cow milkings.

hour MI, over 5 days. Further, and for simplicity of the example, it is assumed that there are 25 cases of CM that all occur on the fifth day of milking. Recall that the disease event to be defined is a mastitis case, or in this case a CM, per cow milking. For each example the prevalence of CM does not alter (25 CM cases per 1000 cow milkings), nor does the sensor system SE (set at 80%).

In **Table 1**, the sensing system SP is 96.9%, resulting in an FAR of 30 per 1000 cow milkings and an SR of 40%. In **Table 2**, the change in sensing system performance is a decrease in SP (from 96.9% down to 94.9%) resulting in an FAR of 50 per 1000 cow milkings and an SR of 29%. In addition, **Table 3** describes an increase in sensor system SP to 98.5% (slightly less than the 99% recommended in ISO 20966). In this scenario the FAR becomes 15 per 1000 cow milkings and an SR of 57%. On first glance, a sensing system SP of 96.9% may seem numerically satisfactory, but the result is 30 cows being flagged for CM assessment by milking staff over 5 days in a herd only milking 100 cows. Even an increase in SP to 98.5% still results in a potentially unacceptable number of cows to be checked. Although there are no farmer-sourced guidelines on what is an acceptable level of false alerts,[63] a survey conducted with 139 Dutch farmers indicated that a low level of false alerts was one of 3 specific considerations when assessing sensor system performance (the other 2 being alerts delivered in a timely way and an emphasis on severe CM cases).[64]

In both the review article by Hogeveen and colleagues[62] and a later review by Rutten and colleagues,[58] the investigators reported that none of the peer-reviewed articles describing AMS sensing system performance claimed results that were equal to, or exceeded, the ISO standard target. Mein and Rasmussen[65] suggested that the SP target described in Annex C[61] is a minimum acceptable level for AMS because it implies 10 false alerts per 1000 cow milkings.

Farmers generally do not check all alerts because of time constraints,[66] so a Dutch study assessed the approach of farm staff incorporating non-AMS information on individual cows to help decide which cows to check for CM.[67] However, the investigators found that the effect of using cow data, by the 12% of farmers who undertook this approach, resulted in only minor improvements in determining true CM cases from false alerts.

Table 3
Same scenario as described in Table 1 but decreased false alert rate

	CM-Positive Cow Milking	CM-Negative Cow Milking	Total
Test Positive	20	15	35
Test Negative	5	960	965
Total	25	975	1000 cow milkings

Sensitivity = 20/25 = 0.80 (80%). Specificity = 960/975 = 0.985 (98.5%). Positive predictive value (SR) = 20/35 = 0.57 (57%). FAR = 10 × (100% − 98.5%) = 15 per 1000 cow milkings.

Defining the Gold Standard

The choice and explanation of any GS used to describe sensor system performance is vital.[58] Annex C in ISO 20966 attempts to deal with methods of detecting abnormal milk and interpretation of test results, and the guideline implies that a true CM case can be defined based on the first few squirts of foremilk. Mein and Rasmussen[65] purport that a more robust approach of defining a CM (or clinical episode) would be clots greater than 2 mm in average diameter persisting for more than 3 squirts of foremilk for at least 2 of 3 consecutive milkings.

Their proposal is supported by reanalysis of New Zealand data from a 650-cow herd monitored for 21 days (26,974 milkings) as part of a study assessing the performance of a novel mastitis sensor system. CM was used as the GS but, depending on the 4 possible interpretations of a true clinical case, the SE of the sensor system ranged from 68% to 88% and the FAR from 3.9 to 7 alerts per 1000 cow milkings. At present, there is no agreement on a suitable GS for CM in AMS research and the situation is compounded by the reality that CM is commonly an infrequent event leading to a weak statistical inference.[65] The requirement for careful assessment of the GS description in any study, combined with the range of sensor types and associated system algorithms, makes comparison of sensor system performance even more complex for farmers or advisers.[62]

Defining the Sensor System Alert Period

A sensor system description should include the sensor alert period or alert window. This period may also be described as the time window of detection[62] or the time resolution of measurement by a sensor to alert.[58] In essence, this describes the time period required for the sensor system (sensor data and associated algorithm) to register a test negative or test positive result; that is, the cow milking is defined by the system as no alert or an alert. In some sensor systems, the initial mastitis alert may be distinguished from a repeated alert at subsequent milkings.

Results from the previously mentioned survey of 139 Dutch farmers supported an ideal alert period of 24 hours only.[64] Hogeveen and colleagues[62] proposed that the alert period should ideally be no longer than 48 hours. With an alert period of 24 to 48 hours, one study found there were no GS episodes of CM with more than a single alert.[60] Although Khatun and colleagues[68] found that altering the alert period with an EC sensor system resulted in only small changes in SP, consensus in the literature indicates that wider alert periods results in increased SR (or positive predictive value) and decreased FAR.[60,63] Hence, alert periods of between 24 and 48 hours, reduce sensor system performance but strike the necessary balance between the workload created by mastitis alert checks by farm staff and the desire to reduce false-positive alerts.

Conceptually, alert period is further explained in **Figs. 1–3**. In all cases, the observed CM episode, or GS detection, is defined as 24 hours (for the purpose of example). In **Fig. 1** the alert period is 48 hours, with both alerts described being classified as false

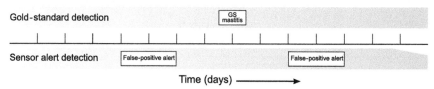

Fig. 1. Relationships between GS detection and sensor system alert detection: 2 false-positive alerts.

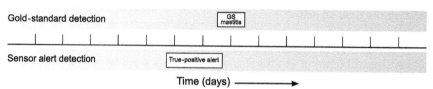

Fig. 2. True-positive alert.

alerts, or false-positive alerts, because they do not overlap with the CM period defined by farmer observation. In **Fig. 2** the alert period is also 48 hours but, in this case, there is overlap between the alert period and the CM period resulting in a true-positive alert (represented in the numerator of the SR calculation). **Fig. 3** shows an alert period of 96 hours (4 days) to make the point that alerts being received by the milking staff at each milking up until the confirmed observation period for CM are likely to result in up to 6 periods in which the cow would be checked without identifying her as having CM and needing treatment.

Electrical Conductivity in Sensor Systems

EC in milk is principally determined by the amount of Na^+ and Cl^- dissolved in the milk,[69] which is normally at a lower concentration compared with blood serum. During inflammation, in the case of subclinical mastitis, or CM, tight junctions of the mammary epithelial cells become leaky, resulting in an increase in Na^+ and Cl^- ions in milk.[70] EC in milk can be affected by factors other than inflammation, such as milk transport, air turbulence, sensor configuration, fat content, and temperature.[71,72]

Various investigators have reported threshold values for EC indicting the presence of mastitis. Hogeveen and Ouweltjes[73] described a threshold for mastitis at 4.6 mS/cm, whereas Hamann and Zecconi[74] described healthy foremilk samples with an EC of 4.9 to 6.4 mS/cm, an EC increase of 0.4 to 1.2 mS/cm in quarters infected with a minor pathogen, and a larger increase to 8 mS/cm in quarters infected with a major pathogen. A fundamental constraint around the use of EC as a single indictor of mastitis is the way the measurement naturally alters during milk let-down.[75] Cisternal milk (milk that has drained into the udder cistern before milk let-down) has an inherently higher EC compared with alveolar milk. Once milk let-down occurs and alveolar milk starts to mix with cisternal milk, EC decreases, with this occurring approximately 40 seconds after the first touch on the udder or teats. Consequently, in AMSs with highly standardized teat-preparation procedures, there is little chance of any milk being tested by a quarter in-line EC sensor being only cisternal in origin. As a consequence of milk let-down, the SE of EC as a mastitis indicator decreases.[44] At present, there exist no guidelines as to the EC threshold to use in AMS for the detection of CM.[68]

Compared with expected changes in ICSCC as a result of a subclinical or clinical infection, the increase in EC is linear, whereas the increase in ICSCC is logarithmic.[71] In AMS, the SE of EC as the primary indicator of mastitis could be improved by

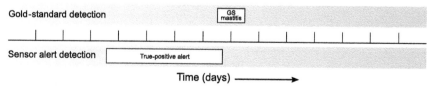

Fig. 3. True-positive alert (wider alert period).

comparing quarters within cow or by comparing repeated measures within cow and between milkings.[66,71] The advantage with quarter measurement is that this comparison can occur within a single milking.[62] Regarding the detection of CM using EC, the range of SE is reported as 47% to 86%, whereas SP ranges from 56% to 99%.[58,68] Various approaches using index creation with EC measurements alone, resulting in suboptimal sensor system performance relative to ISO 20966, has led Khatun and colleagues[68] to conclude that options for using EC for satisfactory CM detection, in isolation from ancillary data in AMS, have been exhausted. Using multiple sensor system information is likely to result in better detection of CM,[76] but not all types of AMS have secondary sensor systems for mastitis detection such as ICSCC.[77] EC probes using 4 probe heads instead of 2 may be more accurate because there is less chance of sensor drift when the EC probes are being used at the quarter level (and between quarter measurements).[66]

Somatic Cell Count (or Proxy Test) in Sensor Systems

Sensor systems that measure (via direct measurement or proxy) ICSCC, or individual quarter SCC, are the other common type of detection system for mastitis in AMS. Sensor systems that use automated counting of stained cell nuclei, based on fluorescence images, have good correlation with laboratory-based measures of SCC; an R^2 of 0.86[78] or up to 0.99.[59] This type of sensor is generally on-line (uses a defined milk sample). A fixed sampling frequency of 24 to 36 hours had the lowest sampling rate in a study reported by Sorensen and colleagues[79] but also the lowest test performance. Sampling frequency is important because of running costs, which have to be taken into account with this sensor type. This finding is in contrast with EC, for which running costs are negligible. In this study, dynamic sampling with a frequency of every 24 hours delivered better test performance and was recommended. The SE was 89% when all data were used but, in practice, IMI alerts may not be practical because of multiple alerts recorded over time.

On-line sensors that perform as automated CMT devices act as a proxy measurement for SCC. The correlation of this sensor system output with laboratory-based SCC is around 0.76 and less when compared with stained cell nuclei methods. Kamphuis and colleagues,[63] when assessing this sensor system for detection of CM, found a 2-fold to 3-fold increase in SR and the same degree of decrease in FAR when a fuzzy logic information system was used in the algorithm creation compared with the use of SCC or EC methods alone.

Color Change in Sensor Systems

In an experiment assessing the degree of blood concentration in milk able to be assessed visually by human test subjects, 0.1% blood in milk was scored as pink (and therefore to be withheld from the bulk tank) when there was reference milk containing no blood for comparison.[80] After this, it was recommended that AMS should be able to detect and divert milk with 100 mg/L blood (0.1%) because, at this level, milk has a red tinge. The combination of EC with sensor information such as color increases mastitis detection system SE and SP where algorithm creation uses fuzzy logic or neural networks.[59]

Incorporation of Other Sensor System or Cow Information

Milking interval change has been postulated as potentially useful information to incorporate into mastitis detection algorithms but the expected increase in MI (decrease in milking frequency) with mastitis has not been reported and so this parameter may not be suitable in AMS.[44] MY losses caused by CM vary according to the month of lactation and can vary from 8% (month 1) through to 1% (month 9) with an average of 5%.[77]

Combining this information into a mastitis detection algorithm in AMSs makes theoretic sense but MY is difficult to predict in a milking system with variable, within-cow, MI.[78,81] Milk production rate may be a more suitable parameter to incorporate into an algorithm for the detection of an IMI.[82]

SUMMARY

In many ways, although the mechanics of milk harvesting in AMS are radically different to conventional milking, the fundamentals of mastitis control in AMSs remain a familiar story to veterinarians, advisers, and dairy farmers. Reducing the amount of teat and udder exposure to environmental material before milking is paramount, as is maintenance of teat health. Reducing the prevalence of teat congestion and teat-end HK are key in this regard. Although assessment of teat health after teat-cup detachment may be more complex in AMSs, the underlying risk factors for this are similar to those of conventional milking.

Diligent and careful consideration of research is required in assessing any given mastitis detection system in AMSs. Although (infrequently published) material on the performance of inflammation enzyme tests has not been addressed in this article, the core questions for an assessment remain the same:

- Can the sensor system be described in the 4 stages from sensor measurement to final advice?
- Is performance reported using robust methods, clear parameters such as SR and FAR, and relative to a well-described GS?

Armed with this information, farmers and their advisers should be in a better position to make valid decisions concerning AMS mastitis detection systems on farms and how they should be applied.

REFERENCES

1. Hallen Sandgren and Emanuelson. Is there an ideal automatic milking system cow and is she different from an ideal parlor-milked cow? 56th Natl. Mastitis Counc. Ann. Mtg. Proc., St. Pete Beach, FL. Natl. Mastitis Counc., New Prague, MN, January 28-31, 2017. p. 61–8.
2. de Koning K, Ouweltjes W. Maximising the milking capacity of an automatic milking system. Wageningen (Netherlands): Wageningen Academic Publishers; 2000.
3. European Union Directive EC/853/2004. 2004.
4. US Food and Drug Adminstration Grade A pasteurized milk ordinance.
5. Hovinen M, Pyörälä S. Invited review: udder health of dairy cows in automatic milking. J Dairy Sci 2011;94:547–62.
6. Rasmussen MD, Blom JY, Nielsen LAH, et al. Udder health of cows milked automatically. Livest Prod Sci 2001;72:147–56.
7. Rasmussen MD. Automatic milking and udder health: an overview. Paris: World Association for Buiatrics; 2006.
8. Hovinen M, Rasmussen MD, Pyorala S. Udder health of cows changing from tie stalls or free stalls with conventional milking to free stalls with either conventional or automatic milking. J Dairy Sci 2009;92:3696–703.
9. Bennedsgaard TW, Elvstrom S, Rasmussen MD. Selection of cows for treatment of udder infections in AMS herds. Wageningen (Netherlands): Wageningen Academic Publishers; 2004.
10. Neave FK, Dodd FH, Kingwill RG. A method of controlling udder disease. Vet Rec 1966;78:521–3.

11. Pankey JW. Premilking udder hygiene. J Dairy Sci 1989;72:1308–12.
12. Barkema HW, Schukken YH, Lam T, et al. Management practices associated with low, medium, and high somatic cell counts in bulk milk. J Dairy Sci 1998;81:1917–27.
13. Schreiner DA, Ruegg PL. Relationship between udder and leg hygiene scores and subclinical mastitis. J Dairy Sci 2003;86:3460–5.
14. Williams DM, Mein GA, Brown MR. Biological responses of the bovine teat to milking: information from measurements of milk flow-rate within single pulsation cycles. J Dairy Res 1981;48:7–21.
15. Hamann J, Mein GA. Teat thickness changes may provide biological test for effective pulsation. J Dairy Res 1996;63:179–89.
16. Reinemann DJ. The smart position on teat condition. Proc. NZ Milk Quality Conference, Hamilton NZ, June 18-19, 2012. p. 141–8.
17. Hamann J, Mein GA. Responses of the bovine teat to machine milking: measurement of changes in thickness of the teat apex. J Dairy Res 1988;55:331–8.
18. Gleeson DE, O'Callaghan EJ, Rath MV. Effect of liner design, pulsator setting, and vacuum level on bovine teat tissue changes and milking characteristics as measured by ultrasonography. Ir Vet J 2004;57:289–96.
19. Bade RD, Reinemann DJ, Zucali M, et al. Interactions of vacuum, b-phase duration, and liner compression on milk flow rates in dairy cows. J Dairy Sci 2009;92:913–21.
20. Mein GA, Brown MR, Williams DM. Pulsation failure as a consequence of milking with short teatcup liners. J Dairy Res 1983;50:249–58.
21. Zecconi A, Bronzo V, Piccinini R, et al. Field study on the relationship between teat thickness changes and intramammary infections. J Dairy Res 1996;63:361–8.
22. Zwertvaegher I, De Vliegher S, Verbist B, et al. Short communication: associations between teat dimensions and milking-induced changes in teat dimensions and quarter milk somatic cell counts in dairy cows. J Dairy Sci 2013;96:1075–80.
23. Countdown Technotes for Mastitis Control, Technote 13, Dairy Australia Publ., Melbourne, Australia.
24. Smart SAMM Technotes, Technote 13, Dairy NZ Publ., Hamilton, NZ.
25. Mein GA Reinemann DJ Making the most of machine on time: what happens when the cups are on? 46th Natl. Mastitis Counc. Ann. Mtg. Proc, San Antonio, TX, January 21-24, 2007. Natl. Mastitis Counc, New Prague, MN. p. 18–30.
26. Upton J, Penry JF, Rasmussen MD, et al. Effect of pulsation rest phase duration on teat end congestion. J Dairy Sci 2016;99:3958–65.
27. Ronningen O, Postma E. Classification of mouthpiece chamber vacuum records in milking-time tests. 51st Natl. Mastitis Counc. Ann. Mtg. Proc., St. Pete Beach FL, January 22-24, 2012. Natl. Mastitis Counc, New Prague, MN. p. 219–20.
28. Penry JF, Upton J, Mein GA, et al. Estimating teat canal cross-sectional area to determine the effects of teat-end and mouthpiece chamber vacuum on teat congestion. J Dairy Sci 2017;100:821–7.
29. Borkhus M, Ronningen O. Factors affecting mouthpiece chamber vacuum in machine milking. J Dairy Res 2003;70:283–8.
30. Neijenhuis F, Barkema HW, Hogeveen H, et al. Classification and longitudinal examination of callused teat ends in dairy cows. J Dairy Sci 2000;83(12):2795–804.
31. Neijenhuis F, Barkema H, Hogeveen H, et al. Relationship between teat-end callosity and occurrence of clinical mastitis. J Dairy Sci 2001;84:2664–72.
32. Mein GA, Williams DMD, Reinemann DJ. Effects of milking on teat-end hyperkeratosis: 1. Mechanical forces applied by the teatcup liner and responses of the teat. National Mastitis Council 2003; Proc. 42nd annual meeting. Fort Worth, Texas, January 26-29, 2003.

33. Mein GA, Reinemann DJ. Biomechanics of milking: teat - liner interactions. Proceedings ASABE Annual International Meeting. June 21-24, 2009.

34. Leonardi S, Penry JF, Tangorra FM, et al. Methods of estimating liner compression. J Dairy Sci 2015;98:6905–12.

35. Mein GA, Neijenhuis F, Morgan WF, et al. Evaluation of Bovine Teat Condition in Commercial Dairy Herds: 1. Non-Infectious Factors. 2nd Int. Symposium on Mastitis and Milk Quality (NMC/AABP) Proc., Vancouver, British Columbia, Canada, September 13-15, 2001. Natl. Mastitis Counc., New Prague, MN. p. 347–351.

36. Dodd FH, Neave FK. Machine milking rate and mastitis. J Dairy Res 1951;18: 240–5.

37. Grindal RJ, Hillerton JE. Influence of milk flow rate on new intramammary infection in dairy cows. J Dairy Res 1991;58:263–8.

38. Brown CA, Rischette SJ, Schultz LH. Relationship of milking rate to somatic-cell count. J Dairy Sci 1986;69:850–4.

39. Halley B, Barlow J, Bramley A, et al. Observational Studies on the Association Between Peak Milk Flow Rate and Somatic Cell Count. 40th Natl. Mastitis Counc. Ann. Mtg. Proc., Reno, NV, February 11-14, 2001. Natl. Mastitis Counc., New Prague, MN. p. 179–180.

40. Hammer JF, Morton JM, Kerrisk KL. Quarter-milking-, quarter-, udder- and lactation-level risk factors and indicators for clinical mastitis during lactation in pasture-fed dairy cows managed in an automatic milking system. Aust Vet J 2012;90:167–74.

41. Penry JF, Crump PM, Ruegg PL, et al. Short communication: cow- and quarter-level milking indicators and their associations with clinical mastitis in an automatic milking system. J Dairy Sci 2017;100:9267–72.

42. Stelwagen K, Phyn CVC, Davis SR, et al. Reduced milking frequency: milk production and management implications. J Dairy Sci 2013;96:3401–13.

43. Klungel GH, Slaghuis BA, Hogeveen H. The effect of the introduction of automatic milking systems on milk quality. J Dairy Sci 2000;83:1998–2003.

44. Fogsgaard KK, Lovendahl P, Bennedsgaard TW, et al. Changes in milk yield, lactate dehydrogenase, milking frequency, and interquarter yield ratio persist for up to 8 weeks after antibiotic treatment of mastitis. J Dairy Sci 2015;98: 7686–98.

45. Dohmen W, Neijenhuis F, Hogeveen H. Relationship between udder health and hygiene on farms with an automatic milking system. J Dairy Sci 2010;93:4019–33.

46. Jago JG, Davis KL, Copeman PJ, et al. The effect of pre-milking teat-brushing on milk processing time in an automated milking system. J Dairy Res 2006;73:187–92.

47. Hovinen M, Aisla AM, Pyorala S. Visual detection of technical success and effectiveness of teat cleaning in two automatic milking systems. J Dairy Sci 2005;88: 3354–62.

48. Knappstein K, Roth N, Walte HG, et al. Effectiveness of automatic cleaning of udder and teats and effects of hygiene management. Report on effectiveness of cleaning procedures applied in different automatic milking systems. Deliverable D14. Automatic Milking, Netherlands. 2004.

49. Bruckmaier RM, Macuhova J, Meyer H. Specific aspects of milk ejection in robotic milking: a review. Livestock Production Science 2001;72(1-2):169–76.

50. Nyhan JF, Cowhig MJ. Inadequate milking machine vacuum reserve and mastitis. Vet Rec 1967;81:122–4.

51. O'Shea, J, and E O'Callaghan. 1978. Milking machine effects on new infection rate. 17th Natl. Mastitis Counc. Ann. Mtg. Proc., Louisville, KY, February 21-23, 1978. Natl. Mastitis Counc., New Prague, MN. p. 262–68.

52. O'Shea J, O'Callaghan E, Meaney B. Liner slips and impacts. Proc. International Mastitis Symposium. Montreal, Canada, 1987. p. 44–65.
53. Thiel CC, Cousins CL, Westgarth DR, et al. The influence of some physical characteristics of the milking machine on the rate of new mastitis infections. J Dairy Res 1973;40:117.
54. Cousins CL, Thiel CC, Westgarth DR, et al. Further short-term studies of the influence of the milking machine on the rate of new mastitis infections. J Dairy Res 1973;40:289.
55. Mein GA, Reinemann DJ. Machine milking and mastitis risk: looking ahead with the benefit of hindsight. 57th Natl. Mastitis Counc. Ann. Mtg. Proc., Tucson, AZ, January 30-February 2, 2018. Natl. Mastitis Counc., New Prague, MN. p. 91–102.
56. Weaver SR, Hernandez LL. Autocrine-paracrine regulation of the mammary gland. J Dairy Sci 2016;99:842–53.
57. Penry JF, Crump PM, Hernandez LL, et al. Association of quarter milking measurements and cow-level factors in an automatic milking system. J Dairy Sci 2018. https://doi.org/10.3168/jds.2017-14153.
58. Rutten CJ, Velthuis AGJ, Steeneveld W, et al. Invited review: Sensors to support health management on dairy farms. J Dairy Sci 2013;96:1928–52.
59. Brandt M, Haeussermann A, Hartung E. Invited review: technical solutions for analysis of milk constituents and abnormal milk. J Dairy Sci 2010;93:427–36.
60. Sherlock R, Hogeveen H, Mein GA, et al. Performance evaluation of systems for automated monitoring of udder health: analytical issues and guidelines. Mastitis Control - from science into practice. Brussels (Belgium): International Dairy Federation; 2008. p. 275–82.
61. International Standards Organization ISO/FDIS 20966, Annex C.
62. Hogeveen H, Kamphuis C, Steeneveld W, et al. Sensors and clinical mastitis–the quest for the perfect alert. Sensors (Basel) 2010;10:7991–8009.
63. Kamphuis C, Sherlock R, Jago J, et al. Automatic detection of clinical mastitis is improved by in-line monitoring of somatic cell count. J Dairy Sci 2008;91: 4560–70.
64. Mollenhorst H, Rijkaart LJ, Hogeveen H. Mastitis alert preferences of farmers milking with automatic milking systems. J Dairy Sci 2012;95:2523–30.
65. Mein GA, Rasmussen MD. Performance evaluation of systems for automated monitoring of udder health: would the real gold standard please stand up? Mastitis Control - from science into practice; 2008. p. 259–66.
66. Claycomb RW, Johnstone PT, Mein GA, et al. An automated in-line clinical mastitis detection system using measurement of conductivity from foremilk of individual udder quarters. N Z Vet J 2009;57:208–14.
67. Steeneveld W, van der Gaag LC, Ouweltjes W, et al. Discriminating between true-positive and false-positive clinical mastitis alerts from automatic milking systems. J Dairy Sci 2010;93:2559–68.
68. Khatun M, Clark CEF, Lyons NA, et al. Early detection of clinical mastitis from electrical conductivity data in an automatic milking system. Anim Prod Sci 2017;57:1226–32.
69. Linzell JL, Peaker M. Efficacy of measurement of electrical-conductivity of milk for detection of subclinical mastitis in cows - detection of infected cows at a single visit. Br Vet J 1975;131:447–61.
70. Stelwagen K, Singh K. The role of tight junctions in mammary gland function. J Mammary Gland Biol Neoplasia 2014;19:131–8.

71. Auldist M. Effect on processing characteristics. Encyclopedia of Dairy Science 2002.
72. Rasmussen MD, Wiking L, Bjerring M, et al. Influence of air intake on the concentration of free fatty acids and vacuum fluctuations during automatic milking. J Dairy Sci 2006;89:4596–605.
73. Hogeveen H, Ouweltjes W. Automatic on-line detection of abnormal milk. Encyclopedia of Dairy Science 2002.
74. Hamann J, Zecconi A. Evaluation of the electrical conductivity of milk as a mastitis indicator. Bulletin 334/1998. Brussels (Belgium): International Dairy Federation; 1998.
75. Bruckmaier RM, Weiss D, Wiedemann M, et al. Changes of physicochemical indicators during mastitis and the effects of milk ejection on their sensitivity. J Dairy Res 2004;71:316–21.
76. Mollenhorst H, van der Tol PP, Hogeveen H. Somatic cell count assessment at the quarter or cow milking level. J Dairy Sci 2010;93:3358–64.
77. Huijps K, Lam T, Hogeveen H. Costs of mastitis: facts and perception. J Dairy Res 2008;75:113–20.
78. Nielsen PP, Pettersson G, Svennersten-Sjaunja KM, et al. Technical note: variation in daily milk yield calculations for dairy cows milked in an automatic milking system. J Dairy Sci 2010;93:1069–73.
79. Sorensen LP, Bjerring M, Lovendahl P. Monitoring individual cow udder health in automated milking systems using online somatic cell counts. J Dairy Sci 2016;99: 608–20.
80. Rasmussen MD, Bjerring M. Visual scoring of milk mixed with blood. J Dairy Res 2005;72:257–63.
81. de Mol RM, Ouweltjes W. Detection model for mastitis in cows milked in an automatic milking system. Prev Vet Med 2001;49:71–82.
82. Kohler SD, Kaufmann O. Quarter-related measurements of milking and milk parameters in an AMS-herd. Milchwissenschaft-Milk Science International 2003; 58:3–6.

Genetic Selection for Mastitis Resistance

Kent A. Weigel, PhD*, George E. Shook, PhD

KEYWORDS

- Dairy cattle • Mastitis • Somatic cell count • Udder health • Genetic selection
- Genomic prediction

KEY POINTS

- Mastitis is the most common and costly disease on most dairy farms, with detrimental impacts including veterinary treatments, lost milk yield, impaired fertility, and premature culling.
- Indirect selection for mastitis resistance using somatic cell count can be effective, and genetic evaluations for somatic cell score (base 2 log transformation of somatic cell count) have been implemented in most countries in the past 25 years.
- Direct selection using clinical mastitis data has been practiced for decades in the Nordic countries, where national veterinary recording systems contain detailed health data from all cows in the population.
- Recently, large-scale genetic and genomic selection programs to improve resistance to mastitis and other common health disorders have been developed using producer-recorded data from herd management software on large commercial farms.

INTRODUCTION

Mastitis has long been a concern of dairy farmers, veterinarians, and animal health professionals worldwide due its impact on health costs, milk yield, milk quality, culling rate, reproductive performance, and, more recently, antibiotic residues and antibiotic resistance. Estimated genetic correlations (r_g) between clinical mastitis (CM) and milk, fat, and protein yields tend to be antagonistic, typically in the range of 0.25 to 0.50, indicating that long-term selection for improved milk production increases the frequency of CM.[1–3] Cows with elevated somatic cell count (SCC) or CM, however, tend to have impaired milk production in the short term, relative to their healthy herd mates, with estimated costs in the range of $0.50 per day to $2.00 per day.[4] Comorbidity with other functional traits, such as early postpartum

Disclosure: The authors have nothing to disclose.
Department of Dairy Science, University of Wisconsin–Madison, 1675 Observatory Drive, Madison, WI 53706-1205, USA
* Corresponding author.
E-mail address: kweigel@wisc.edu

health, fertility, and longevity, is another concern. Mastitis affects a cow's ability to achieve and maintain pregnancy, and it leads to a 2-fold to 4-fold increase in the risk of premature culling.[5–7]

The overarching goal of dairy farming is to produce healthy and nutritious dairy products for the consumer, but mastitis has negative effects on the shelf life and processing characteristics of milk. For example, Finnish Ayrshire cows that were genetically predisposed to high SCC tended to produce milk with longer coagulation time, higher noncoagulation rate, and reduced curd firmness.[8] Improving environmental conditions and management practices, such as bedding cleanliness and milking hygiene, should be the first priority in reducing mastitis prevalence. Improvement of mastitis resistance through genetic selection, however, can provide permanent gains, which may lessen dependence on antibiotic treatments and reduce the risk of antibiotic-resistant bacterial strains.[9,10]

Approximately 70 years ago, heritable genetic variation in the incidence of mastitis was demonstrated, suggesting the possibility of genetic selection for improved mastitis resistance in dairy cattle.[11] Subsequent investigators established strong genetic correlations between CM, bacteriologic status, and SCC.[12,13] These studies laid the foundation for genetic improvement programs targeting udder health. A comprehensive review outlined priorities and strategies for using genetic selection to improve dairy cow health, noting that undesirable correlated responses to selection for milk yield necessitate the inclusion of health traits in the breeding goal.[14] The investigator concluded that breeding for resistance to mastitis and other diseases was justified economically, but closer cooperation was needed to incorporate genetics in the veterinary medicine curriculum and integrate veterinary data into milk recording programs. Three decades later, such cooperation and integration has not been realized, at least in North America. This review focuses on opportunities for achieving permanent improvements in mastitis resistance through genetic and genomic selection. Other investigators have also provided excellent reviews of strategies for genetic improvement of mastitis resistance in dairy cattle.[15]

Glossary of genetic terms
  Heritability (h^2): the proportion of observed variation in a trait that can be attributed to genetic differences between individuals or families
  Breeding value (BV): the genetic superiority or inferiority of a particular animal, relative to the average of the population. The BV reflects an animal's genetic contribution to its own observation or measurement for the trait.
  Estimated BV (EBV): a statistical estimate of the BV, computed from measurements of the trait taken on the animal, its ancestors, and its offspring
  Genomic EBV (GEBV): an EBV that has been augmented with information from genomic testing using a commercially available DNA microarray
  Transmitting ability (TA): the genetic superiority or inferiority that a particular animal passes to its progeny, relative to the average of the population. The TA reflects the animal's genetic contribution its offspring's observation or measurement for the trait. Note that TA = ½ BV.
  Predicted TA (PTA): a statistical estimate of the TA, computed from measurements of the trait taken on the animal, its ancestors, and its offspring. Note that PTA = ½ EBV.
  Genomic PTA (GPTA): a PTA that has been augmented with information from genomic testing using a commercially available DNA microarray. Note that GPTA = ½ GEBV.

Reliability (REL): an estimate of the accuracy of an EBV, GEBV, PTA, or GPTA, ranging from 0.00 (random guess) to 0.99 (nearly perfect), calculated by counting the information available from ancestors, progeny, own performance, and genomic testing

Genetic correlation (r_g): a measure of the extent to which an animal's genetic superiority or inferiority for 1 trait predisposes that animal to genetic superiority or inferiority in a second trait, ranging from -1.00 (perfectly negative relationship) to 0.00 (no relationship) to $+1.00$ (perfectly positive relationship)

SELECTION BASED ON SOMATIC CELL SCORE

Since the early 1980s, SCC has been measured in monthly milk samples of individual cows in Dairy Herd Improvement (DHI) milk recording programs as an aid to management of mastitis at the herd and individual cow levels. Although somatic cells include both epithelial cells and white blood cells, a majority of variations between cows and among repeated tests from the same cow are caused by immune cells that migrate into milk in response to a mastitis infection.

Converting Somatic Cell Count to Somatic Cell Score

The frequency distribution of SCC has 2 undesirable characteristics that are detrimental, in terms of statistical analysis and interpretation of results:

- Mean SCC is often substantially greater than median SCC.
- SCC lacks the familiar bell-shaped normal curve; instead, there are high frequencies of samples with low SCC and increasingly scarce frequencies of samples with high SCC.

Statistical properties of test-day SCC were examined, with the finding that a logarithmic transformation was nearly ideal among a large family of transformations.[16] In the early 1980s, a base 2 log (log_2) transformation was adopted to transform SCC to somatic cell score (SCS).[17] This transformation is used by milk recording programs in the United States, Canada, and many other countries. Advantages of a log_2 transformation, in comparison to a natural log (ln) or base 10 log transformation, are

- A 1-point increase (or decrease) in SCS translates to doubling (or halving) of SCC.
- The range of scores is greater, suggesting greater importance of the trait.

Regardless of the base, all log transformations result in

- SCS values that are approximately normally distributed
- Mean SCS that closely approximates the median SCS within a herd or population
- Higher h^2 estimates for SCS (0.12) than SCC (0.06)[18]
- Greater statistical power in hypothesis testing[19]

Formula for converting SCC (in cells/µL) to SCS:

$$SCS = log_2 (SCC/100) + 3 = \ln (SCC/100)/\ln (2) + 3 = \ln (SCC/100)/0.6931 + 3$$

For example, SCC 400 translates to SCS 5.

Formula for converting SCS to SCC (cells/µL) or mean SCS to geometric mean SCC:

$$SCC = 100 \times 2^{(SCS - 3)} = 100 \times e^{[(SCS - 3) \times \ln (2)]} = 100 \times e^{[(SCS - 3) \times 0.6931]}$$

For example, SCS 5 translates to SCC 400.

Heritability and Genetic Correlation Estimates for Somatic Cell Score and Clinical Mastitis

To establish the validity of genetic selection for lower SCS, it was essential to demonstrate that SCS is heritable and that it has a strong genetic correlation with CM. Estimates of h^2 and r_g parameters from 3 countries are shown in **Table 1**.

In other studies, h^2 estimates in Dutch Meuse-Rhine-Issel cattle and United States Holsteins were 0.08 and 0.10, respectively.[23,24] Estimated r_g of SCS with CM have been reported in 3 other populations: Danish Holsteins (0.97), Norwegian Reds (0.62), and United States Holsteins (0.67).[25–27] Also, a Dutch study found that daughters of bulls with high progeny versus low progeny means for SCS in first lactation differed significantly in SCS and percentage of infected quarters during later lactations.[23]

In summary, results show that h^2 estimates are greater for SCS than CM, meaning that predictions of genetic merit of cows and bulls are determined more accurately from SCS. Also, high estimates of the r_g between SCS with CM indicate that SCS can be used successfully to achieve genetic improvement in mastitis resistance.

Phenotypic Relationship of Somatic Cell Score with and Intramammary Infection

A logistic regression model was used to assess the relationship between SCS and probability of intramammary infection (IMI) (assessed using bacterial culture) between 120 days and 305 days postpartum.[28] A 1-unit increase in SCS increased the odds of IMI by 84%. Recently, the relationship between SCS and IMI was examined with 79,308 cows in 1124 dairy herds in the northeastern United States.[29] Each 1-point increase in SCS was associated with a 2.3%, 5.5%, and 9.1% increase in prevalence of contagious IMIs, environmental IMIs, and all IMIs, respectively. Furthermore, the investigators concluded that the relationship between SCS and IMI was stable across demographic variables, such as year, season, housing system, herd size, parity, stage of lactation, and use or nonuse of a coliform mastitis vaccine.

National and International Genetic Evaluation for Somatic Cell Score

In the United States, adjustment factors for parity, stage of lactation, and season were developed to combine test-day SCS into a lactation measure.[30] And in 1994, national genetic evaluations for SCS were implemented in the United States.[24,31] This was the first concerted attempt to improve the health of North American dairy cattle through genetic selection. At the time, CM data were unavailable for most herds, but SCC data were collected routinely for approximately 80% of herds in a DHI milk recording

Table 1
Estimates of heritability for somatic cell score, clinical mastitis, and intramammary infection and genetic correlation of somatic cell score with clinical mastitis or intramammary infection in diverse dairy populations

Country	Heritability of Clinical Mastitis or Intramammary Infection	Heritability of Somatic Cell Score	Genetic Correlation of Somatic Cell Score with Clinical Mastitis or Intramammary Infection
Sweden CM[20]	0.05	0.08	0.60
Israel CM[21]	0.01	0.27	0.30
Israel IMI[21]	0.05	0.27	0.99
France CM[22]	0.02	0.17	0.72

program, and PTA for SCS were computed in the same manner as PTA for milk production traits.

National genetic evaluations for SCS were developed and implemented in Canada as well.[32,33] The Canadian implementation focused on the advantages of using a test-day model to account for month-to-month fluctuations in udder health, as opposed to simply averaging SCS across the whole lactation. Procedures were developed at Interbull (Uppsala, Sweden) to extend within-country genetic evaluations for SCS (12 countries) and CM (3 Nordic countries only) to an international scale.[34] Estimates of the r_g between CM in Nordic countries and SCS in non-Nordic countries had a median of 0.55, indicating that selection of dairy sires for semen importation using SCS information is likely to confer improvement in resistance to CM as well. These international evaluations of foreign animals are shared with contributing countries and subsequently combined with in-country evaluations, thereby increasing REL.

Incorporating Somatic Cell Score into Selection Indexes

Selection indexes combine genetic evaluations for several traits into a single measure of total economic merit that farmers can use to make breeding decisions involving specific animals. Traits are weighted by their economic values, and economic weights for SCS consider costs, such as veterinary treatments, discarded milk, and reduced milk yield. A simulation approach was used to evaluate selection programs with and without inclusion of SCS in the breeding goal.[35] The investigators concluded the rate of increase in CM over time could be reduced by 20% to 25%, with only a 1% to 2% reduction in the rate of improvement for yield traits, resulting in a 1% increase in total economic merit. A restricted index, however, that allowed no increase in CM would reduce genetic progress by up to 27% for yield traits and 17% for overall economic merit. Using assumed economic values, the investigators concluded that simultaneous improvement of yield traits and mastitis resistance was not economically justified, due to higher h^2 and greater economic value of yield traits; however, the rate of increase in CM could be slowed considerably by incorporating SCS into a national selection index.

Other Approaches to Using Somatic Cell Score in Genetic Improvement

Efforts to improve genetic evaluations for mastitis resistance and understand the implications of selecting for lower SCS continued in subsequent years. A study of genetic relationships between levels of herd-average SCS concluded that evidence for significant sire by management level interactions (a type of genotype by environment interaction), were lacking.[36] Consequently, genetic evaluations for SCS should include data from herds of all management levels, and separate evaluations for herds with high average SCS and low average SCS are unnecessary. In another study using data from Swedish Holsteins, the investigators found strong genetic correlations between first, second, and third lactations for CM (>0.70) and SCS (>0.80), suggesting that both observations of udder health could be treated as repeated measures of the same biological trait across lactations.[37]

The question of whether cows with low early SCSs are more or less susceptible to CM in later lactation was addressed in a Finnish Ayrshire population.[38] Approximately half of CM cases occurred in the first 8 weeks postpartum (53% and 46%, respectively, in first and second parity cows), whereas the incidence of CM throughout the remainder of lactation decreased gradually. Estimated r_g of CM with SCS before and after the CM episode were 0.69 and 0.69, respectively, in first parity cows, and 0.70 and 0.59, respectively, in second parity cows. This indicates that CM and SCS are strongly correlated, but evidence is lacking that cows with low initial SCS are more likely to experience CM than cows with high initial SCS.

Some investigators have tried to develop proxies for CM using SCC data. Traits, such as proportion of test-day SCC greater than 150,000 cells/mL, presence or absence of test days with SCC greater than,250,000 cells/mL, and number of consecutive test days with SCC greater than,150,000, were examined as alternatives to monthly or lactation average SCS.[39] h^2 estimates for these alternatives, however, were not substantially different from those of conventionally defined SCS, and r_g between all traits were 0.70 or higher.

Alternatives to Somatic Cell Score

Three studies considered other milk composition traits as predictors of IMI. In 1 study, lactose content, SCC, log SCC, and log N-acetyl-B-D-glucosaminidase activity were used to predict IMI status of dairy cows.[19] Log SCC was most useful for differentiating cows with or without IMI, whereas log NAGase was useful for discriminating between major and minor pathogens. In a recent Swedish study, investigators compared log transformations of SCC, lactate dehydrogenase, and NAGase for detecting IMI, and sensitivity and specificity were greatest for ln SCC.[40] The potential for using electrical conductivity (EC) as a mastitis indicator was also considered.[41] Differences in EC reflect changes in concentrations of Na^+, K^+, and Cl^- in milk due to breakdown of tight junctions in mammary epithelial cells during infection. A potential advantage of EC is that it can be measured in the parlor at every milking, whereas SCS data are typically recorded for only 1 or 2 milkings per month. Heritability (h^2) estimates of EC were moderate, ranging from 0.12 to 0.36, whereas r_g between EC and CM ranged from 0.65 to 0.80. These results suggest strong potential for improvement of mastitis resistance through indirect selection based on EC. Systems for pooling quarter-level EC data across farms, validating data quality and completeness, and computing sire EBV and cow EBV, however, are lacking at present.

Genetic and Phenotypic Trends for Somatic Cell Score

Overall, breed average SCS of sire identified US Holstein and Red and White cows on DHI test has decreased from 3.17 for cows born in 1990 to 2.32 for cows born in 2015; these SCSs translate to median SCC values of 112,000 cells/mL and 62,000 cells/mL.[42] This improvement in mastitis resistance is due to changes in both management and genetics, and genetic trends for SCS for United States Holsteins are shown in **Fig. 1**. Although genetic evaluations for SCS became available in 1994, EBV for SCS continued to increase until 2001. This delay can be largely attributed to the aforementioned negative r_g between SCS and milk production, as well as a slow adoption rate by dairy farmers and sire analysts and a relatively small weight for SCS in the national selection index. Since 2001, EBV have decreased steadily, and the rate of decrease has become greater in recent years. The recent acceleration in genetic progress may be due to genomic testing of young bulls and cows (since 2009) as well as increased focus on improving health traits. In Canada, the average EBV for SCS decreased by 0.15 points from 2004 to 2014, translating to a 10% decrease in the geometric mean of SCC.[43]

Although the reduction in average SCS has been accomplished primarily by improved herd management, selection for lower SCS has been effective in improving udder health. These genetic gains are permanent, and gains accumulate from one generation to the next. Nevertheless, augmenting selection for lower SCS with direct selection using CM data could provide additional improvements, provided that such data can be collected in a cost-effective manner.

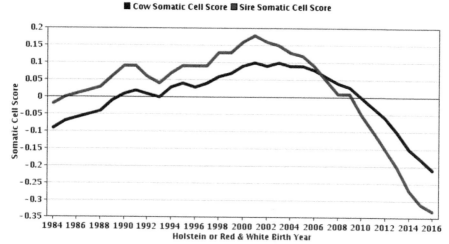

Fig. 1. Genetic trend for SCS in United States Holstein cows and bulls, by year of birth. (*Courtesy of* Council on Dairy Cattle Breeding, Bowie, MD; with permission).

SELECTION USING VETERINARIAN OR PRODUCER-REPORTED MASTITIS DATA

As discussed previously, much of the work on genetic selection for improved mastitis resistance, and improved health of dairy cattle in general, was pioneered in the Nordic countries.[44] Norwegian farmers, academics, and veterinarians noticed an increase in the number of veterinary treatments per 100 cows as early as the 1960s, and they developed a comprehensive health recording system that formed the basis of genetic selection programs for improved dairy cow health in Norway as well as much of the scientific literature on genetic selection for resistance to mastitis.

In another early study, h^2 of CM was estimated as 0.12 using CM records from 24 commercial farms in southern England.[45] In Danish Red cattle, h^2 estimates were 0.054, 0.056, and 0.059 for CM from 10 days prepartum to 50 days, 180 days, and 350 days postpartum, respectively.[46] By comparison, estimated h^2 from 50 days to 180 days postpartum, 180 days to 350 days postpartum, and 50 days to 350 days postpartum were 0.0007, 0.0002, and 0.020, respectively. Therefore, the investigators recommended that selection should focus on CM in early lactation. In another study using data of more than 470,000 Danish Holstein cows, the h^2 estimate was 0.035 for CM between 10 days prepartum and 50 days postpartum.[47]

In Norway, an increase of 13% to 28% was reported in observed CM incidence from 15 days prepartum to 120 days postpartum during the period from 1978 through 1994, and h^2 of CM was estimated as 0.029.[48] In a subsequent study, the investigators divided the lactation into 11 intervals of 30 days and analyzed CM on a monthly basis with a threshold model that accounted for the binary nature of incidence data.[49] And at the genetic level, the trend in average EBV for CM of Norwegian cows born from 1976 to 1990 using the more sophisticated model was nearly flat (−0.02% per year) and a more substantial rate of improvement (−0.27% per year) was observed in recent years, suggesting that selection for reduced CM is becoming more effective over time.[50] In a subsequent Swedish study, a survival analysis model was used to account for cows that were culled from the herd prior to completing the "opportunity period" for CM, and this led to higher h^2 estimates (0.03–0.04) than a linear model (0.01–0.02).[51] In a German study, CM incidence was based on veterinary treatment records, whereas subclinical mastitis was assessed using the California mastitis test, and h^2 estimates were 0.06 for CM and 0.03 for subclinical mastitis.[52] Lastly, in a recent Swedish study, genetic trends for SCS and CM from 1990 to 2007 were neutral or slightly unfavorable, despite efforts to improve mastitis resistance in the Nordic countries.[53]

In the United States, data from on-farm herd management software on commercial dairies were used to estimate h^2 and predict sire PTA for CM and other health traits.[54] Heritability estimates for CM were 0.07 and 0.06 in the first lactation and all lactations, respectively, and the predicted lactational incidence rate of CM was 2-fold higher among daughters of the worst sires, compared with daughters of the best sires. The investigators concluded that, in the absence of a national veterinary recording system, genetic improvement of CM and other health disorders is possible using producer-reported incidence data from on-farm herd management software programs, as long as herd-year-season contemporary groups are large enough to permit side-by-side comparisons of the offspring of different sires under the same management, diagnostic, and reporting conditions. A later study considered the incidence of CM in different lactations as well as in different periods of the same lactation as separate traits in a multitrait model.[55] The investigators concluded that genetic correlations between lactations, although moderate (0.42–0.49), tended to be higher than correlations between distant points in the same lactation (0.24–0.64), particularly when comparing early lactation with mid-lactation or late lactation. Sire PTA for the probability of no reported cases of CM in first lactation ranged from 0.77 to 0.89, whereas sire PTA for the probability of no reported cases of CM during the first 3 lactations ranged from 0.36 to 0.59.

Recently, a genomic component was added to the aforementioned work by using incidence data from on-farm herd management software to estimate genetic parameters of CM using pedigree-based and genomic prediction models.[27,56] The investigators also evaluated the accuracy of genomic predictions using cross-validation. Heritability estimates for liability to CM ranged from 0.05 to 0.11, whereas estimates for SCS ranged from 0.08 to 0.18. The REL of sire PTA for CM from the pedigree-based analysis was only 0.16, on average, but average REL increased to 0.54 when SCS data were incorporated using a bivariate model. Adding genomic data provided additional gains in REL of sire GPTA for CM, with average REL values of 0.68 and 0.80 in the univariate and bivariate analyses, respectively.

The first implementation of genetic or genomic predictions for common health disorders of dairy cattle in United States, by Zoetis Genetics (Kalamazoo, Michigan), included mastitis, metritis, retained placenta, displaced abomasum, ketosis, and lameness.[57] Their analysis combined more than 100,000 single nucleotide polymorphism (SNP) genotypes, with 14 million pedigrees and 4 million performance records for the incidence of CM from on-farm herd management software of commercial farms. Average REL of the GPTA for young selection candidates for CM was 52%, and the introduction of genomic predictions for CM and other common health disorders in 2016 enabled United States dairy farmers to select for improved health and wellness in their cattle. Recently, the Council on Dairy Cattle Breeding (Bowie, Maryland) implemented national genetic evaluations for CM, hypocalcemia, displaced abomasum, ketosis, metritis, and retained placenta in United States dairy cattle using similar methodology.[56]

Additional developments in genomic prediction methods, in particular, electronic data capture systems, will enable more advancements in selection for mastitis resistance. For example, data from Danish Holstein cows in automatic milking systems with inline SCC measurement were used to evaluate a cow's risk of mastitis (transition from healthy to diseased state) as well as her ability to recover from mastitis (transition from diseased state to healthy state).[58] Heritability estimates for mastitis risk and recovery rate were 0.07 and 0.08, respectively, and the estimated r_g between risk and recovery was strongly negative (−0.83), indicating that cows with high risk for CM infection generally take significantly longer to recover from the CM infection. This study, among others, demonstrates the power of routine electronic data capture systems to study not only the incidence of mastitis and other important diseases but also the trajectory of progression and recovery for each disease or disorder.

SELECTION FOR SPECIFIC GENOMIC REGIONS OR VARIANTS

As described previously, pedigree-based selection for mastitis resistance has given way to genomic selection using dense SNP genotype data for all chromosomes. Depending on the genetic architecture of the trait, however, marker-assisted selection for specific quantitative trait loci (QTL) or known genetic variants may be an alternative. Variants in genes encoding bovine lactoferrin and lysozyme were characterized as possible candidates for the improvement of mastitis resistance through selection or creation of transgenic dairy cows.[59] Even at that time, when modern tools for genetic manipulation had not yet been developed, the investigators lamented the challenge of identifying candidate genes affecting mastitis susceptibility in populations of dairy cattle that lack detailed phenotypes for CM and related traits. Nonetheless, their vision for applying modern biotechnologies in the context of bovine mastitis became reality when transgenic cows were produced that resisted *Staphylococcus aureus* challenge via secretion of small amounts of lysostaphin in their milk.[60] More recently, it was reported that milk of transgenic cows created by inserting the human lysozyme gene into the β-casein locus had the ability to kill *S aureus* pathogens.[61]

Transgenic cattle bring ethical and consumer considerations, and selection for specific variants is possible by other means if knowledge about their effects on mastitis resistance is available. Significant associations were reported between udder health and class I and class II alleles of the bovine major histocompatibility complex (BoLA) in Simmental and Simmental × Red Holstein dairy cattle.[62] Later, significant differences in allelic frequencies were found at the *BoLA-DRB3.2* locus between lines of Norwegian Red cattle selected for low CM or high protein yield, a result that could be caused by either selection or drift.[63] In that study, 2 associations were confirmed in the broader Norwegian Red cow population. The investigators concluded that future studies should focus on *BoLA* haplotypes rather than single genes, but they noted that genes in the *BoLA-DRB* group account for only a small proportion of the difference in CM between the selection lines.

A genome-wide association study, using data from German Holstein bulls, found that 16 SNPs and 10 haplotype blocks were associated with variation in SCS.[64] Previously reported QTL on chromosomes 5, 6, 18, and 19 were confirmed in this study, with allele substitution effects of up to 14,000 cells/mL. The investigators noted that minor (low-frequency) alleles associated with lower SCS on chromosomes 18 and 19 are of particular interest for genomic selection. Data from Danish Holstein sires were used to evaluate contributions of specific genetic markers to biological pathways associated with SCS and CM that occurred early (15 days prepartum to 50 days postpartum) or late (51–305 days postpartum) in first lactation.[65] Biological pathways associated with carbohydrate metabolism and the excretory system explained variation in mastitis in early lactation; however, the proportion of variance in udder health due to these pathways was far less than that of milk, fat, or protein yield. Other investigators attempted fine-mapping of QTL for milk yield and CM on *Bos taurus* autosome 20.[66] The strongest associations between candidate mutations for CM and milk yield were more than 3.5 megabases apart, suggesting that it should be possible to break antagonistic genetic correlations between production traits and udder health using genomic selection.

Medium-density (54,000) and imputed high-density (777,000) SNP panels were compared with imputed whole-genome sequence data for the detection of QTL associated with udder health.[67] In this study, udder health was defined as the Danish index that combines CM in early first, late first, second, and third lactations with weights of 0.25, 0.25, 0.30, and 0.20, respectively. Greater marker density enhanced statistical power for detection of QTL and refinement of chromosomal location, and the investigators identified 33 candidate QTL regions that were associated with udder health. A genome-wide expression analysis was carried out using primary bovine mammary gland epithelial cells derived from cows with favorable or unfavorable alleles for a QTL on chromosome 18 that is known to be associated with SCS.[68] Cells from cows with the favorable QTL allele had a faster and stronger response to *Escherichia coli* and *S aureus* challenge, compared with cells from cows carrying the unfavorable allele. Also, a QTL was fine-mapped on bovine chromosome 6 and identified a 12-kilobase duplication in an exon of the group-specific component (GC) gene near SNP markers that were associated with increased mastitis susceptibility.[69] This mutation has not yet been associated, however, with RNA expression and protein levels of the GC gene during mastitis infection.

Recently, it was proposed to incorporate biological knowledge from the functional annotation of genomes into whole-genome selection programs by preferentially weighting SNPs or genomic regions that are likely to contain causal mutations.[70] This approach was applied to CM data of Nordic Holstein and Jersey cows. The genomic variance of CM was not distributed evenly across all chromosomes but rather enriched in a subset of hepatic transcriptomic regions that responded to IMI with *E coli*, as quantified by RNA sequencing. Incorporating biological knowledge into this approach improved the accuracy of genomic predictions relative to conventional genomic methods. The performance of these methods will improve in the future, as the quality and quantity of functional annotation of the bovine genome improve. Another study evaluated the relationship between copy number variation and EBV of Holstein sires for SCS.[71] More than 2 dozen copy number variations were associated with SCS, and candidate genes in networks related to stress, cell death, inflammation, and immune response were identified.

SELECTION FOR GENERAL IMMUNE FUNCTION

Genetic and genomic selection programs for improved udder conformation, lower SCS, and reduced incidence of CM have been developed, as have selection programs for reduced incidence of other common health disorders. In general, cows that are more susceptible to infection by 1 type of mastitis pathogen also tend to be more susceptible to infection by another. Also, for example, cows that are genetically predisposed to one type of early postpartum health disorder tend to have increased risk of another. This raises the question of whether measures of general immune function that might simultaneously reduce the incidence or severity of mastitis and other health disorders could be selected for. A quarter century ago, lactating Holstein cows were evaluated using a battery of standard immune function assays; the investigators found differences between sire progeny groups in lymphocyte blastogenesis and various measures of neutrophil function, several of which were associated with differences in SCC.[72] The investigators concluded that genetic variation exists between families in nonspecific humoral and cellular immunity.

Later investigators studied the relationships of SCS, CM, and IMI due to major pathogens with molecular markers at the IgG2, DRB3, and CD18 loci as well as physiologic measures of immune function during the periparturient period from 35 days prepartum to 35 days postpartum.[73] Allele substitution effects were significantly associated with CM at all 3 loci. In addition, sire EBV for various immune function assays, such as mononuclear cell activity, stimulated chemiluminescence, random migration, IgG1, ingestion, and cytochrome C reduction were significantly associated (in a positive or negative manner) with EBV for SCS, CM, and major-pathogen IMI, suggesting the possibility of selection for general immune function as a way to increase mastitis resistance.

Differences have been reported in cell-mediated immune response (CMIR) and antibody-mediated immune response (AMIR) in Canadian Holstein cows using delayed-type hypersensitivity and serum antibody tests, respectively.[74] Heritability estimates were 0.19 for CMIR and 0.16 to 0.41 for AMIR, depending on time interval and test antigen, suggesting the possibility of selection for adaptive immune response and overall disease resistance. In a related study, Holstein cows were classified as high, average, or low for CMIR, AMIR, and overall immune response, and the investigators noted higher incidence of CM among cows that were classified as average compared with cows that had high values for AMIR, CMIR, or overall IR.[75] Subsequently, this group reported that cows with high AMIR had an incidence rate for CM of 0.17 cases per cowyear compared with 0.28 for cows with average AMIR and 0.31 for cows with low AMIR.[76] In addition, severity of CM tended to be greater for cows with low AMIR. No differences were found, however, between cows classified as high, average, or low for CMIR, which the investigators attributed to the extracellular nature of mastitis pathogens. Additional research is needed to confirm associations between measures of immune function and the incidence of CM and other common health disorders as well as to elucidate cause-effect relationships. These studies provide insight, however, into the interrelationships between immune function, mastitis incidence, and mastitis severity.

SUMMARY

The animal breeding and genetics literature from the past 3 decades is rich with studies of SCS, CM, and related measures of udder health. Foundational work in the Nordic countries later spread to continental Europe and North America. Today, nearly every leading dairy country has a national evaluation system that ranks bulls and cows based on their genetic evaluation for SCS. Furthermore, genetic or genomic improvement programs that use CM data from national veterinary databases or producer-reported CM data from on-farm herd management software are becoming common. The incidence and severity of mastitis are influenced heavily by environmental conditions and management practices. Regardless, significant genetic variation exists among families, and this can be used to confer permanent improvement in mastitis resistance. When EBVs for SCS and CM are incorporated into selection indexes, producers can improve the production potential of their cattle for milk solids, while also improving genetic resistance to CM and other common health disorders or at least minimizing the impact of antagonistic genetic relationships between health and yield traits. Future studies will further elucidate the biological pathways that contribute to mastitis resistance or susceptibility as well as its severity and the cow's ability to recover fully. In addition, it is likely that knowledge of specific genetic variants that contribute to mastitis resistance will be used in selection and mating decisions. Possibilities for using such information in conjunction with techniques such as gene editing will depend on governmental policies and consumer acceptance.

Take-home suggestions for practicing veterinarians:

- Recognize that genetic variation exists between cows in mastitis resistance, and sire selection can contribute to long-term improvement of herd health.
- Genetic evaluations for SCS have been available for more than 20 years, and selection of sires with PTA or GPTA values less than 3.00 will reduce SCC in the next generation.
- Genomic predictions for mastitis resistance are now available, and selection of sires with Council on Dairy Cattle Breeding GPTA values greater than 0.00 or Zoetis GPTA values greater than 100 will reduce the incidence of CM in future generations.
- Sire selection decisions will be most effective when using measures of overall profit, such as the Council on Dairy Breeding Lifetime Net Merit Index or the Zoetis Dairy Wellness Profit Index.

REFERENCES

1. Heringstad B, Chang YM, Gianola D, et al. Genetic association between susceptibility to clinical mastitis and protein yield in Norwegian dairy cattle. J Dairy Sci 2005;88:1509–14.
2. Hinrichs D, Stamer E, Junge W, et al. Genetic analyses of mastitis data using animal threshold models and genetic correlation with production traits. J Dairy Sci 2005;88:2260–8.
3. Negussie E, Strandén I, Mantysaari EA. Genetic association of clinical mastitis with test-day somatic cell score and milk yield during first lactation of Finnish Ayrshire cows. J Dairy Sci 2008;91:1189–97.
4. Hadrich JC, Wolf CA, Lombard J, et al. Estimating milk yield and value losses from increased somatic cell count on US dairy farms. J Dairy Sci 2018;101: 3588–96.
5. Weller JI, Ezra E. Genetic analysis of somatic cell score and female fertility in Israeli Holsteins with an individual animal model. J Dairy Sci 1997;80:586–93.
6. Caraviello DZ, Weigel KA, Shook GE, et al. Assessment of the impact of somatic cell count on functional longevity in Holstein and Jersey cattle using survival analysis methodology. J Dairy Sci 2015;88:804–11.
7. Roxström A, Strandberg E. Genetic analysis of functional, fertility-, mastitis-, and production-determined length of productive life in Swedish dairy cattle. Livest Prod Sci 2002;74:125–35.
8. Ikonen T, Morri S, Tyriseva A-M, et al. Genetic and phenotypic correlations between milk coagulation properties, milk production traits, somatic cell count, casein content, and pH of milk. J Dairy Sci 2004;87:458–67.
9. Moon J-S, Lee A-R, Kang H-M, et al. Phenotypic and genetic antibiogram of methicillin-resistant Staphylococci isolated from bovine mastitis in Korea. J Dairy Sci 2007;90:1176–85.
10. Frey Y, Rodriguez JP, Thomann A, et al. Genetic characterization of antimicrobial resistance in coagulase-negative staphylococci from bovine mastitis milk. J Dairy Sci 2013;96:2247–57.
11. Lush JL. Inheritance of susceptibility to mastitis. J Dairy Sci 1950;33:121–5.
12. Legates JE, Grinnells CD. Genetic relationships in resistance to mastitis in dairy cattle. J Dairy Sci 1952;35:829–33.
13. Young CW, Legates JE, Lecce JG. Genetic and phenotypic relationships between clinical mastitis, laboratory criteria, and udder height. J Dairy Sci 1960; 43:54–62.

14. Shook GE. Selection for disease resistance. J Dairy Sci 1989;72:1349–62.
15. Martin P, Barkema HW, Bitro LF, et al. *Symposium review:* novel strategies to genetically improve mastitis resistance in dairy cattle. J Dairy Sci 2018;101: 2724–36.
16. Ali AKA, Shook GE. An optimum transformation for somatic cell concentration in milk. J Dairy Sci 1980;63:487–90.
17. Shook GE. Genetic improvement of mastitis through selection on somatic cell count. Vet Clin North Am Food Anim Pract 1993;9:563–81.
18. Monardes HG, Kennedy BW, Moxley JE. Heritabilities of measures of somatic cell count per lactation. J Dairy Sci 1983;66:1707–13.
19. Berning LE, Shook GE. Prediction of mastitis using milk somatic cell count, N-acetyl-B-D-glucosaminidase, and lactose. J Dairy Sci 1992;75:1840–8.
20. Emanuelson U, Dannell B, Philipsson J. Genetic parameters for clinical mastitis, somatic cell counts, and milk production estimated by multiple-trait restricted maximum likelihood. J Dairy Sci 1988;71:467–76.
21. Weller JI, Saran A, Zeliger Y. Genetic and environmental relationships among somatic cell count, bacterial infection, and clinical mastitis. J Dairy Sci 1992;75: 2532–40.
22. Rupp R, Boichard B. Genetic parameters for clinical mastitis, somatic cell score, production, udder type traits, and milking ease in first lactation Holsteins. J Dairy Sci 1999;82:2198–204.
23. Vecht U, Shook GE, Politiek RD, et al. Effect of bull selection for somatic cell count in first lactation in cell counts and pathogens in later lactations. J Dairy Sci 1985; 68:2995–3003.
24. Schutz MM. Genetic evaluation of somatic cell scores for United States dairy cattle. J Dairy Sci 1994;77:2113–29.
25. Lund MS, Jensen J, Petersen PH. Estimation of genetic and phenotypic parameters for clinical mastitis, somatic cell production deviance, and protein yield in dairy cattle using Gibbs sampling. J Dairy Sci 1999;82:1045–51.
26. Heringstad B, Gianola D, Chang YM, et al. Genetic associations between clinical mastitis and somatic cell score in early first-lactation cows. J Dairy Sci 2006;89: 2236–44.
27. Parker Gaddis KL, Tiezzi F, Cole JB, et al. Genomic prediction of disease occurrence using producer-recorded health data: a comparison of methods. Genet Sel Evol 2015;47:41–53.
28. Rodriguez-Zas SL, Gianola D, Shook GE. Bayesian analysis via Gibbs sampling of susceptibility to intramammary infection in Holstein cattle. J Dairy Sci 1998;81: 2710–22.
29. Shook GE, Bamber Kirk RL, Welcome FL, et al. Relationship between intramammary infection prevalence and somatic cell score in commercial herds. J Dairy Sci 2017;100:9691–701.
30. Wiggans GR, Shook GE. A lactation measure of somatic cell count. J Dairy Sci 1987;70:2666–72.
31. Shook GE, Schutz MM. Selection on somatic cell score to improve resistance to mastitis in the United States. J Dairy Sci 1994;77:648–58.
32. Reents R, Dekkers JCM, Schaeffer LR. Genetic evaluations for somatic cell score with a test day model for multiple lactations. J Dairy Sci 1995;78:2858–70.
33. Reents R, Jamrozik J, Schaeffer LR, et al. Estimation of genetic parameters for test day records of somatic cell score. J Dairy Sci 1995;78:2847–57.
34. Mark T, Fikse WF, Emanuelson U, et al. International genetic evaluations of Holstein sires for milk somatic cell and clinical mastitis. J Dairy Sci 2002;85:2384–92.

35. Strandberg E, Shook GE. Genetic and economic responses to breeding programs that consider mastitis. J Dairy Sci 1989;72:2136–42.

36. Banos G, Shook GE. Genotype by environment interaction and genetic correlations among parities for somatic cell count and milk yield. J Dairy Sci 1990;73:2563–73.

37. Carlén E, Strandberg E, Roth A. Genetic parameters for clinical mastitis, somatic cell score, and production in the first three lactations of Swedish Holstein cows. J Dairy Sci 2004;87:3062–70.

38. Koivula M, Mantysaari EA, Negussie E, et al. Genetic and phenotypic relationships among milk yield and somatic cell count before and after clinical mastitis. J Dairy Sci 2005;88:827–33.

39. de Haas Y, Ouweltjes W, ten Napel J, et al. Alternative somatic cell count traits as mastitis indicators for genetic selection. J Dairy Sci 2008;91:2501–11.

40. Nyman A-K, Emanuelson U, Persson Waller K. Diagnostic test performance of somatic cell count, lactate dehydrogenase, and N-acetyl-β-D glucosaminidase for detecting dairy cows with intramammary infection. J Dairy Sci 2016;99:1440–8.

41. Norberg E. Electrical conductivity of milk as a phenotypic and genetic indicator of bovine mastitis: a review. Livest Prod Sci 2005;96:129–39.

42. Council on Dairy Cattle Breeding. Trend in somatic cell score for holstein and red & white. Available at: https://queries.uscdcb.com/eval/summary/trend.cfm. Accessed April 23, 2018.

43. Canadian Dairy Network. National genetic trends by birth year for Holstein cows. Available at: https://www.cdn.ca/files_ge_articles.php. Accessed April 25, 2018.

44. Solbu H. Disease recording in Norwegian dairy cattle I. Disease incidences and non-genetic effects on mastitis, ketosis, and milk fever. Z Tierzuecht Zuechtungsbiol 1983;100:139–57.

45. Bunch KJ, Heneghan DJS, Hibbitt KG, et al. Genetic influences on clinical mastitis and its relationship with milk yield, season, and stage of lactation. Livest Prod Sci 1984;11:91–104.

46. Lund T, Miglior F, Dekkers JCM, et al. Genetic relationships between clinical mastitis, somatic cell count, and udder conformation in Danish Holsteins. Livest Prod Sci 1994;39:243–51.

47. Hansen M, Lund MS, Sørensen MK, et al. Genetic parameters of dairy character, protein yield, clinical mastitis, and other diseases in the Danish Holstein cattle. J Dairy Sci 2002;85:445–52.

48. Heringstad B, Klemetsdal G, Ruane J. Clinical mastitis in Norwegian cattle: Frequency, variance components, and genetic correlation with protein yield. J Dairy Sci 1999;82:1325–30.

49. Heringstad B, Chang YM, Gianola D, et al. Genetic analysis of longitudinal trajectory of clinical mastitis in first-lactation Norwegian cattle. J Dairy Sci 2003a;86:2676–83.

50. Heringstad B, Rekaya R, Gianola D, et al. Genetic change for clinical mastitis in Norwegian cattle: a threshold model analysis. J Dairy Sci 2003b;86:369–75.

51. Carlén E, Schneider P, Strandberg E. Comparison between linear models and survival analysis for genetic evaluation of clinical mastitis in dairy cattle. J Dairy Sci 2005;88:797–803.

52. Gernand E, Rehbein P, von Borstel UU, et al. Incidences of and genetic parameters for mastitis, claw disorders, and common health traits recorded in dairy cattle contract herds. J Dairy Sci 2012;95:2144–56.

53. Eriksson S, Johansson K, Hansen Axelsson H, et al. Genetic trends for fertility, udder health, and protein yield in Swedish Red cattle estimated with different models. J Anim Breed Genet 2017;134:308–21.

54. Zwald NR, Weigel KA, Chang YM, et al. Genetic selection for health traits using producer-recorded data. I. Incidence rates, heritability estimates, and sire breeding values. J Dairy Sci 2004;87:4287–94.

55. Zwald NR, Weigel KA, Chang YM, et al. Genetic analysis of clinical mastitis data from on-farm management software using threshold models. J Dairy Sci 2006;89: 330–6.

56. Parker Gaddis KL, Cole JB, Clay JS, et al. Genomic selection for producer-recorded health events in US dairy cattle. J Dairy Sci 2014;97:3190–9.

57. Vukasinovic N, Bacciu N, Przybyla CA, et al. Development of genetic and genomic evaluation for wellness traits in US Holstein cows. J Dairy Sci 2017; 100:428–38.

58. Welderufael BG, Janss LLG, de Koning DJ, et al. Bivariate threshold models for genetic evaluation of susceptibility to and ability to recover from mastitis in Danish Holstein cows. J Dairy Sci 2017;100:4706–20.

59. Seyfert H-M, Henke M, Interthal H, et al. Defining candidate genes for mastitis resistance in cattle: the role of lactoferrin and lysozyme. J Anim Breed Genet 1996;113:269–76.

60. Wall RJ, Powell AM, Paape MJ, et al. Genetically enhanced cows resist intrammammary Stapylococcus aureus infection. Nat Biotechnol 2005;23:445–51.

61. Liu X, Wang Y, Tian Y, et al. Generation of mastitis resistance in cows by targeting human lysozyme gene to β-casein locus using zinc-finger nucleases. Proc Biol Sci 2014;281(1780):20133368.

62. Arriëns MA, Ruff G, Schällibaum M, et al. Possible association between a serologically detected haplotype of the bovine Major Histocompatibility Complex and subclinical mastitis. J Anim Breed Genet 1994;111:152–61.

63. Kulberg S, Heringstad B, Guttersrud OA, et al. Study on the association of *BoLa-Drb3.2* alleles with clinical mastitis in Norwegian Red cows. J Anim Breed Genet 2007;124:201–7.

64. Abdel-Shafy H, Bortfeldt RH, Tetens J, et al. Single nucleotide polymorphism and haplotype effects associated with somatic cell score in German Holstein cattle. Genet Sel Evol 2014;46:35–44.

65. Edwards SM, Thomsen B, Madsen P, et al. Partitioning of genomic variance reveals biological pathways associated with udder health and milk production traits in dairy cattle. Genet Sel Evol 2015;47:60–72.

66. Kadri NK, Guldbrantsen B, Lund MS, et al. Genetic dissection of milk yield traits and mastitis resistance quantitative trait loci on chromosome 20 in dairy cattle. J Dairy Sci 2015;98:9015–25.

67. Wu X, Lund MS, Sahana G, et al. Association analysis for udder health based on SNP-panel and sequence data in Danish Holsteins. Genet Sel Evol 2015;47: 50–63.

68. Brand B, Hartmann A, Repsilber D, et al. Comparative expression profiling of *E. coli* and *S. aureus* inoculated primary mammary gland cells sampled from cows with different genetic predispositions for somatic cell score. Genet Sel Evol 2011;43:24–40.

69. Olsen HG, Knutsen TM, Lewandowska-Sabat AM, et al. Fine mapping of a QTL on bovine chromosome 6 using imputed full sequence data suggests a key role for the *group-specific component (GC)* gene in clinical mastitis and milk production. Genet Sel Evol 2016;48:79–94.

70. Fang L, Sahana G, Ma P, et al. Exploring the genetic architecture and improving genomic prediction accuracy for mastitis and milk production traits in dairy cattle by mapping variants to hepatic transcriptome regions responsive to intra-mammary infection. Genet Sel Evol 2017;49:44–61.

71. Durán Aguilar M, Román Ponce SI, Ruiz López FJ, et al. Genome-wide association study for milk somatic cell score in Holstein cattle using copy number variation as markers. J Anim Breed Genet 2017;134:49–59.

72. Kehrli ME Jr, Weigel KA, Freeman AE, et al. Bovine sire effects on daughters' in vitro blood neutrophil functions, lymphocyte blastogenesis, serum complement, and conglutinin levels. Vet Immunol Immunopathol 1991;27:303–19.

73. Kelm SC, Detilleux JC, Freeman AE, et al. Genetic association between parameters of innate immunity and measures of mastitis in periparturient Holstein cattle. J Dairy Sci 1997;80:1767–75.

74. Thompson-Crispi KA, Sewalem A, Miglior F, et al. Genetic parameters of adaptive immune response traits in Canadian Holsteins. J Dairy Sci 2012;95:401–9.

75. Thompson-Crispi KA, Hine B, Quinton M, et al. Short communication: association of disease incidence and adaptive immune response in Holstein dairy cows. J Dairy Sci 2012;95:3888–93.

76. Thompson-Crispi KA, Miglior F, Mallard BA. Incidence rates of clinical mastitis among Canadian Holsteins classified as high, average, or low immune responders. Clin Vaccine Immunol 2013;20:106–12.

Impact and Mitigation of Heat Stress for Mastitis Control

Geoffrey E. Dahl, PhD

KEYWORDS

• Season • Host response • Dry period • Cooling

KEY POINTS

- Heat stress abatement is not difficult to implement, and at a minimum all cows should have shade access regardless of housing or pasture access.
- Active cooling of lactating cows and dry cows can have dramatic effects on productive function and enhance immune status as well; whereas the method of abatement may vary depending on humidity conditions at a particular location, cooling can be achieved in any environment.
- Producers should emphasize appropriate heat stress abatement throughout the production cycle to improve productivity and health, including limiting mastitis.

HEAT STRESS DEFINED

Heat stress occurs when an animal's ability to rid the body of heat is exceeded and body temperature exits the thermoneutral zone (TNZ). In mature cattle the TNZ is from −15°C to 25°C, a clear indication that cows are better able to cope with lower temperatures than upper temperatures in the environment. This circumstance is particularly a problem for mature, lactating cows because of heat generated by the rumen during feed digestion. Indeed, one of the first visible signs of heat stress is a reduction in dry matter intake in cows, in an effort to reduce the internal heat load. Cows will also increase water intake under heat stress and may increase standing time in an effort to maximize heat loss.[1] All of these outcomes will reduce the energy status of a cow by shifting nutrient use to unproductive processes.

Environmental temperatures greater than the TNZ will lead to heat stress, but elevated humidity of an environment exacerbates the effect of temperature. Because cows rid the body of heat primarily through evaporative mechanisms at higher temperatures, elevated humidity will reduce the flow of water and, thus, heat away from the

Research support from NSF (Award #1247362) and USDA-NIFA (Award #2015-67015-23409) gratefully acknowledged.
Department of Animal Sciences, Institute of Food and Agricultural Sciences, University of Florida, Gainesville, FL 32611, USA
E-mail address: gdahl@ufl.edu

Vet Clin Food Anim 34 (2018) 473–478
https://doi.org/10.1016/j.cvfa.2018.07.002
0749-0720/18/© 2018 Elsevier Inc. All rights reserved.

cow to the environment. Therefore, a combination of a relatively milder temperature with high humidity can still cause significant heat stress. A temperature-humidity index (THI) is often used to more accurately reflect the true impact of the environment on the cow. Whereas rectal or vaginal temperatures are often used to assess heat stress in controlled studies, the respiration rate is a simple, accurate indicator of heat stress in cattle as well. Observation of flank movements for 30 to 60 seconds in a sample of cows in a pen or lot is an easy, effective measure of the relative heat stress, with values greater than 60 breaths per minute (bpm) a threshold of heat stress; respiration rates of 75 to 80 bpm are not uncommon in cows in the absence of active cooling.

ENDOCRINE EFFECTS RESULTING FROM HEAT STRESS

Circulating cortisol is an indicator of many stress responses, and cows are no different; but alterations in adrenal output may vary with time as heat stress progresses. Initially, there is an acute increase in cortisol as temperatures increase, but chronically there is a decrease in cortisol as animals adapt to the elevated heat load.[1] This shift in adrenal tone likely affects immune function. Indeed, heat stress caused an increase in circulating leukocyte counts in a similar manner to direct corticotrophin injection in lactating cows, supporting the concept of a linkage between endocrine and immune function.[2] Of interest, a parallel increase in somatic cell count (SCC) was observed in response to heat stress and corticotrophin, indicating that circulating leukocytes could serve as a proxy for mammary gland level immune status.

Prolactin (PRL) is another endocrine signal of the immune system and is considered a cytokine.[3] Many stressors and environmental signals will alter PRL signaling, either via secretion or through receptor expression; these include photoperiod, heat stress, and psychosocial stressors.[3] Relative to cooled animals, with heat stress, circulating PRL increases and receptor expression will decrease in a normal negative feedback accommodation.[4] There is also evidence that immune function is negatively impacted when PRL responsiveness is depressed, as with the decrease in PRL receptor under heat stress and long days.[4,5] Collectively the effects of heat stress on cortisol and PRL are consistent with a decrease in cow immune function.

HEAT STRESS IMPACTS ON MILK QUALITY AND QUANTITY

Using somatic cell scores or counts as an indicator of udder health, several studies have identified heat stress as a contributor to lower milk quality. For example, Zeinhom and colleagues[6] examined SCC and yield on a single farm under extreme THI conditions over 1 year. Under THI ranging from less than 72 to greater than 78, milk SCC was elevated as THI increased and milk fat and protein declined. Pathogen loads increased with THI, as total coliform counts and fecal coliforms were higher at a THI greater than 78 and isolation of *Staphylococcus aureus* and *Escherichia coli* increased with greater THI.

Lambertz and colleagues[7] tracked the acute effects of variable THI increments across 5 commercial herds using test-day records over a 1-year period. Increases in THI from 60 to greater than 65 in the 3 days preceding a test were associated with increases in SCS. Milk yield and composition were similarly decreased, with fat corrected milk and fat and protein percentage all reduced when THI increased.

Nasr and El-Tarabany[8] examined test-day records of cows in a subtropical environment across variable THI values. Similar to other studies, when THI increased, a concomitant increase in SCC was observed. Further, milk yield and composition were inversely related to THI, with lower total milk, fat, and protein percentages and yield at the highest THI.

HEAT EFFECTS ON MASTITIS ORGANISMS
In Vitro Studies

Lecchi and colleagues[9] isolated polymorphonuclear cells from healthy midlactation cows and exposed them to hyperthermic conditions in vitro. After 2 hours at 41°C, polymorphonuclear neutrophils (PMNs) had lower phagocytosis and oxidative burst capacity compared with those incubated at 39°C, indicating a direct reduction in the capacity of immune cells to respond to pathogens. In contrast, Elvinger and colleagues[10] also cultured PMNs from cows in vitro at 38.5°C and 42.0°C but observed no effect of hyperthermia on phagocytosis or killing of E coli. However, lymphocyte proliferation was reduced with long-term (60 hours) incubation at high temperatures but that reduction was less in lymphocytes collected from cows under heat stress in vivo. Thus, the duration of the heat stress may affect immune cell responses, and heat stress may induce adaptive responses that allow lymphocytes to survive longer.

Lactating Cows

Although there are limited data regarding the direct effect of heat stress alone on mastitis, several studies have found a relationship between intramammary infection incidence and season, with the general assumption being that hotter seasons are more conducive to pathogen growth; thus, exposure to the cow will increase in the summer months. However, recent reports suggest a more nuanced relationship among season, pathogen, and cow factors likely exists.

Lundberg and colleagues[11] followed 13 herds in Sweden over a 12-month period to identify relationships among pathogen, herd, season, and parity on udder infection in early lactation. All the herds followed had suboptimal udder health. Whereas mastitis was generally more prevalent in the summer months relative to cooler times, this was not the case for all pathogens. For example, Streptococcus dysgalactiae infection rates were highest at the end of the summer pasture season, when cows would have been under heat stress. In contrast, Streptococcus uberis infection rates peaked at the end of the housing season during the winter. Finally, S aureus infection rates varied among herds; but there was little relationship to season. These data suggest that although some increase in pathogen load may appear with hotter temperatures, other factors are also influencing intramammary infection rates.

Gao and colleagues[12] assessed the mastitis pathogen prevalence in 161 large dairy herds in China over an 18-month period and determined the seasonal factors affecting those pathogens causing clinical mastitis. Clinical mastitis was increased during the summer, which was associated with higher prevalence of E coli and Klebsiella spp. In contrast, S dysgalactiae, other streptococci, and S agalactiae were more frequently isolated in the winter. Thus, there is no consistent pathogen predominance across seasons or geographic locations, further suggesting that cow factors are a significant contributor to the development of mastitis in warmer weather.

Dry Cows

Several recent studies have examined the impact of heat stress on immune function in dry cows, with a subsequent determination of the relative effect on performance and health in the next lactation. Similar to lactating cows, heat-stressed dry cows reduce dry matter intake; but in contrast to lactating cows, there is no evidence of altered basal insulin, glucose, or nonesterified fatty acids (NEFA) in circulation.[13] Nor is there any change in response to insulin or glucose challenge under heat stress in dry cows, although residual responses are apparent following parturition.[13] However, those shifts in glucose, NEFA, and responses to insulin postpartum are consistent with the observed effects of heat stress on mammary output and, thus, not directly linked to heat stress.

Both adaptive and innate immune function are altered by heat stress in the dry cow model but differ with regard to timing and direct induction by heat stress. do Amaral and colleagues[4] observed that heat stress depressed lymphocyte proliferation relative to cooled dry cows. In addition, heat stress reduced immunoglobulin G output in response to an immunization with ovalbumin, suggesting that vaccination responses may be affected under conditions of heat stress.[14] After calving, lymphocytes from previously heat-stressed cows had altered the expression of several genes related to immune status. Specifically, there were residual effects of dry period heat stress to depress the PRL receptor and increase suppressors of cytokine signaling, indicating a shift in PRL responsiveness related to reduced immune function.[4] Early in lactation, circulating tumor necrosis factor alpha was elevated in cows that were cooled during the dry period, which is likely to have implications for immune responsiveness during the transition.[4]

Residual impacts on innate immune function are also apparent with dry period heat stress. During the dry period, no differences were observed in phagocytosis or oxidative burst capacity with heat stress or cooling, yet after parturition cows cooled when dry had a greater circulating neutrophil number[14] and higher oxidative burst and phagocytic action relative to cows that experienced heat stress when dry. It is important to note that the improved innate immune function was coincident with elevations in circulating NEFA and β-hydroxybutyrate, typically a situation whereby a reduction in immune status would be expected.[15]

Limited controlled evidence exists to suggest that dry period heat stress reduces the cow's ability to respond to pathogens in lactation, but at least 2 studies support that concept. Using cows that experienced heat stress when dry, the authors challenged them at 5 days in milk (DIM) with *S uberis* in one-quarter and saline in the opposite quarter and monitored the development of mastitis and other outcomes for the next 72 hours.[16] Prepartum cooling resulted in greater circulating neutrophil numbers and improved responses to *S uberis* relative to cows that had been under heat stress before calving. It is important to emphasize that during the challenge, all cows had access to active cooling, so the response was a carryover from the dry period treatment.

But does heat stress in the dry period alter disease incidence in the next lactation? To test that hypothesis, the authors compared cows that were dry during the hottest (ie, June, July, August) months of the year with herd mates that were dry in the coolest months of the year (December, January, and February). The records were obtained from a large commercial dairy with very consistent feeding, housing, and general management; the groups were of similar genetic potential.[17] When dry, all cows were housed on pasture without any structural shade beyond trees. As in controlled studies, cows that were dry in the cooler months produced more milk in the next lactation. Of more interest, cows dry during the cooler months had a reduced incidence of mastitis, respiratory disease, and retained fetal membranes, all outcomes consistent with improved immune function.

HEAT STRESS ABATEMENT

Given the forgoing discussion of the negative impacts of heat stress on lactating and dry dairy cattle, it is of interest to consider how best to reduce the heat load in a normal housing situation on farms (reviewed in Ref.[1]). Shade is the first approach to consider, at a minimum, as the reduction in radiant heat can have dramatic effects on heat accumulation in the cow housed on pasture or in an open lot. The shade area should provide a minimum of 19 ft^2 of space for each cow, but that may increase as the severity of heat stress increases and the density of cows under the shade has to decrease. And it is wise to account for the angle of the sun when installing shades to maximize the effective shading throughout the afternoon.

The next step is active cooling, usually a combination of soaking cows with water and then using fans to move air over the cows and improving water movement from the cows' skin to the environment and heat along with that water during evaporation. When this process is repeated throughout the day, very effective cooling of lactating and dry cows is possible. Another technique is to cool the air around the cows by using water to carry heat from the air as misted water evaporates. Combined with air movement via fans, this approach works especially well in drier, arid environments, as the evaporation of water can be maximized relative to more humid conditions.

Another consideration is the location of the cooling and the priority of cooling by production stage. Holding pen cooling is important in the milking string, as that location is one where cows can accumulate a significant heat load and will be exposed to that insult 2 or 3 times each day. In typical free stall barns, soakers can be installed over the feed line and fans can then be placed over stalls. With that approach, cows will be soaked with water when feeding and that water will be evaporated as they lay in the stalls, effectively providing active cooling regardless of the stage of lactation. However, this approach minimizes the contamination of stall beds with water, which reduces the chances of increased pathogen growth.

SUMMARY

Although there are limited numbers of controlled studies that have examined the impact of heat stress on mastitis, the evidence available suggests that the concept that higher mastitis incidence in summer is not a simple outcome of greater pathogen loads. Indeed, the physiologic effects of heat stress on both lactating and dry cows cause reductions in immune competence that can persist for extended periods and suppress the response to pathogen exposure, which then exacerbates the higher pathogen exposure, leading to greater mastitis.

Heat stress abatement is not difficult to implement, and at a minimum all cows should have shade access regardless of housing or pasture access. Active cooling of lactating cows and dry cows can have dramatic effects on productive function and enhance immune status as well. Whereas the method of abatement may vary depending on humidity conditions at a particular location, cooling can be achieved in any environment. Therefore, producers should emphasize appropriate heat stress abatement throughout the production cycle to improve productivity and health, including limiting mastitis.

REFERENCES

1. Collier RJ, Dahl GE, VanBaale MJ. Major advances associated with environmental effects on dairy cattle. J Dairy Sci 2006;89:1244–53.
2. Wegner TN, Schuh JD, Nelson FE, et al. Effect of stress on blood leucocyte and milk somatic cell counts in dairy cows. J Dairy Sci 1976;59:949–56.
3. Dahl GE. Effects of short day photoperiod on prolactin signaling in dry cows: a common mechanism among tissues and environments? J Anim Sci 2008;86(13 Suppl):10–4.
4. do Amaral BC, Connor EE, Tao S, et al. Heat stress abatement during the dry period influences prolactin signaling in lymphocytes. Domest Anim Endocrinol 2010;38:38–45.

5. Auchtung TL, Dahl GE. Prolactin mediates photoperiodic immune enhancement: effects of administration of exogenous prolactin on circulating concentrations, receptor expression, and immune function in steers. Biol Reprod 2004;71:1913–8.

6. Zeinhom MM, Abdel Aziz RL, Mohammed AN, et al. Impact of seasonal conditions on quality and pathogens content of milk in Friesian cows. Asian-Australas J Anim Sci 2016;29:1207–13.

7. Lambertz C, Sanker C, Gauly M. Climatic effects on milk production traits and somatic cell score in lactating Holstein-Friesian cows in different housing systems. J Dairy Sci 2014;97:319–29.

8. Nasr MA, El-Tarabany MS. Impact of three THI levels on somatic cell count, milk yield and composition of multiparous Holstein cows in a subtropical region. J Therm Biol 2017;64:73–7.

9. Lecchi C, Rota N, Vitali A, et al. In vitro assessment of the effects of temperature on phagocytosis, reactive oxygen species production and apoptosis in bovine polymorphonuclear cells. Vet Immunol Immunopathol 2016;182:89–94.

10. Elvinger F, Hansen PJ, Natzke RP. Modulation of function of bovine polymorphonuclear leukocytes and lymphocytes by high temperature in vitro and in vivo. Am J Vet Res 1991;52:1692–8.

11. Lundberg Å, Nyman AK, Aspán A, et al. Udder infections with Staphylococcus aureus, Streptococcus dysgalactiae, and Streptococcus uberis at calving in dairy herds with suboptimal udder health. J Dairy Sci 2016;99:2102–17.

12. Gao J, Barkema HW, Zhang L, et al. Incidence of clinical mastitis and distribution of pathogens on large Chinese dairy farms. J Dairy Sci 2017;100:4797–806.

13. Tao S, Thompson IM, Monteiro APA, et al. Effect of cooling heat-stressed dairy cows during the dry period on insulin response. J Dairy Sci 2012;95:5035–46.

14. do Amaral BC, Connor EE, Tao S, et al. Heat stress abatement during the dry period influences metabolic gene expression and improves immune status in the transition period of dairy cows. J Dairy Sci 2011;94:86–96.

15. do Amaral BC, Connor EE, Tao S, et al. Heat-stress abatement during the dry period: does cooling improve transition into lactation? J Dairy Sci 2009;92: 5988–99.

16. Thompson IM, Tao S, Monteiro AP, et al. Effect of cooling during the dry period on immune response after Streptococcus uberis intramammary infection challenge of dairy cows. J Dairy Sci 2014;97:7426–36.

17. Thompson IM, Dahl GE. Dry period seasonal effects on the subsequent lactation. Prof Anim Sci 2012;28:628–31.

Methods for Diagnosing Mastitis

Pamela R.F. Adkins, DVM, PhD*, John R. Middleton, DVM, PhD

KEYWORDS

• Bovine • Mastitis • Intramammary infection • Diagnosis

KEY POINTS

- The most common cause of mastitis is an intramammary infection.
- Considering cost and ease of data collection, somatic cell count is the most common diagnostic test used for the detection of subclinical mastitis.
- Bacteriologic culture and polymerase chain reaction are the primary methods currently in use to diagnose intramammary infection.
- There is no gold standard for the diagnosis of mastitis or intramammary infection.

INTRODUCTION

Mastitis is defined as inflammation of the mammary gland. The most common cause of mastitis is an intramammary infection (IMI). An IMI refers to the presence of an infectious organism in the mammary gland. Although these two often go hand in hand and the terms are frequently used interchangeably, no single diagnostic test is able to define both. A diagnosis of mastitis is generally based on measuring the inflammatory response, whereas diagnosis of an IMI is based on identification of the inciting infectious agent. Diagnosis of mastitis by measuring indicators of inflammation is often used as an indirect method to identify cows with an IMI.

DIAGNOSIS OF MASTITIS
Clinical Mastitis

Mastitis can be characterized as clinical or subclinical. Clinical mastitis is defined as visibly abnormal milk from a mammary quarter. With forestripping, that is, visual examination of a stream of milk collected immediately before routine milking, clinical mastitis can easily be detected (**Fig. 1**). Clinical mastitis can be defined based on severity as mild, moderate, or severe.[1] Severity scoring systems can be used to determine appropriate treatment and the risk of an undesirable outcome.[2]

Disclosure Statement: The authors have nothing to disclose.
Department of Veterinary Medicine and Surgery, University of Missouri, 900 East Campus Drive, Columbia, MO 65211, USA
* Corresponding author.
E-mail address: adkinsp@missouri.edu

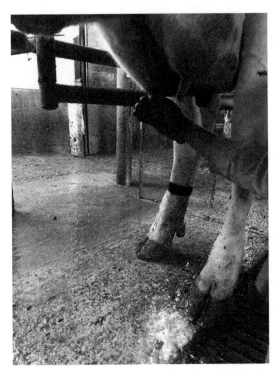

Fig. 1. Forestripping can help to identify cases of clinical mastitis in the parlor.

- Mild clinical mastitis: Abnormal milk only (usually manifest by clots, flakes, and/or changes in the color and consistency of the milk secretion).
- Moderate clinical mastitis: Abnormal milk and abnormal mammary gland (manifest by inflammatory changes in the tissue such as redness, heat, pain, and swelling).
- Severe clinical mastitis: Abnormal milk, abnormal mammary gland, and sick cow (manifest by changes in body temperature, rumination rate, appetite, hydration status, and demeanor).[2]

Subclinical Mastitis

Subclinical mastitis is defined as the presence of inflammation with a normal appearing mammary gland and visibly normal milk. Many tests have been evaluated for the diagnosis of subclinical mastitis. Some of the more common ones are listed here.

- Somatic cell count (SCC): Concentration of leukocytes (primarily) per milliliter of milk. Leukocytes comprise 80% of the somatic cells in uninfected quarters and 99% in infected quarters.[3] The most important factor that causes a rise in SCC is an IMI.
- Lactose: The percentage of lactose in mastitic milk is lower. This change occurs owing to tissue damage causing decreased synthetic ability of the enzyme systems in the secretory cells, resulting in reduced lactose biosynthesis.[4]
- Lactate dehydrogenase (LDH): An enzyme found in most tissues, including the cytoplasm of leukocytes. When cell damage occurs, to either mammary epithelial cells or leukoctyes, LDH is released into the milk.[4] Some commercially available mastitis detection tools incorporate measurement of LDH activity.

- N-acetyl-β-ᴅ-glucosaminidase (NAGase): A lysosomal enzyme that is released into the milk from damaged mammary epithelial cells and, to a lesser extent, from milk somatic cells.[5,6]
- Acute phase proteins: Haptoglobin and milk amyloid A have been found in milk owing to their migration from blood into milk across the blood–milk barrier because of increased capillary permeability and loss of tight junctions, or through local production by milk leukocytes or mammary epithelial cells.[7]
- Conductivity: Electrical conductivity (EC) of milk increases with mastitis owing to an increase in sodium and chloride concentrations and a decrease in the potassium concentration.[4] Several milking equipment manufacturers have used EC as an in-line method of detecting mastitis.

Somatic Cell Count

Taking cost and ease of data collection into consideration, SCC or the logarithmic transformation of SCC, the somatic cell score (SCS), is the most common diagnostic test used for the detection of subclinical mastitis. In a laboratory setting, SCC can be measured using microscopy, referred to as direct microscopic SCC or by using automated electronic cell counters. The direct microscopic SCC method is performed by spreading a specific volume of milk within a calibrated area of a microscopic slide. After the milk dries, the slide is stained, and visible cells are counted within the defined area. The method is labor intensive, requires a high-quality microscope, and necessitates thorough training of personnel to gain proficiency. Automated electronic cell counters, which commonly are based on flow cytometric methods, allow for rapid and easy determination of SCC. Creameries, Dairy Herd Information Association, and other dairy organizations use automated electronic cell counters, making these data highly accessible. Portable counters are also available and can be used to test SCC in the laboratory or on the farm.

At the herd level, SCC data are generally available on every shipment of milk that leaves the farm and these data provide an estimation of overall udder health among cows contributing to the bulk tank milk. At the cow level, herds that use a testing laboratory such as the Dairy Herd Information Association, generally have monthly data reflecting the udder health of each cow, and these data can be used in parallel to predict which cows have healthy mammary glands versus those with acute, resolved, or chronic cases of subclinical mastitis (**Fig. 2**).

Although cow-level composite SCC samples are useful for separating infected from uninfected cows, these data are imperfect. The sensitivity of composite SCC as an indicator for IMI in at least one-quarter ranges from 30% to 89%, whereas the specificity ranges from 60% to 90%.[8–10] The sensitivity and specificity using a threshold of 200,000 cells/mL for a single composite SCC obtained closest to the time of culture were 44% and 87%, respectively, for cows infected with any pathogen and 65% and 73%, respectively, for cows infected with major pathogens.[10]

The most accurate relationship between IMI and SCC exists at the quarter level. Data suggest that uninfected quarters have a mean SCC of approximately 70,000 cells/mL[11,12] and an SCC of 200,000 cells/mL or greater or an SCS of 4 or higher is often used as a threshold to define infected quarters.[11] That said, diagnostic sensitivity of quarter-level SCC for subclinical mastitis can also be imperfect, and somewhat depends on the pathogen inciting the mastitis. Middleton and colleagues[13] reported that sensitivity of quarter-level SCC using a threshold of 100,000 cells/mL (SCS = 3) was 0.60 for all bacterial IMI, 0.53 for coagulase negative staphylococcal IMI, 0.96 for coagulase positive staphylococcal IMI, and 0.71 for IMI with non-*agalactiae Streptococcus*-like organisms.

Other limitations have been identified that impact the use of SCC as a diagnostic tool. Milk SCC can remain elevated for some time after an organism has been eliminated, resulting in a false-positive test for IMI. Also, although IMI is the predominant factor associated with variation in the SCC, other factors can affect the SCC including herd, cow, breed, quarter, month of sampling, season, stage of lactation, age of the cow, parity, frequency of milking, and stressors.[14–17]

Estimating the Somatic Cell Count at the Cow Side

A number of cow-side methods have been developed and studied for counting or approximating milk SCC.

- California mastitis test (CMT): A qualitative measurement of SCC. The reagent causes lysis of cell membranes and precipitation of the cell DNA and proteins resulting in change in viscosity of the reagent when added to milk.
- Wisconsin mastitis test (WMT): A modification of the CMT developed to increase the objectivity of measuring the viscosity. A modification of the WMT has been adapted for on-farm use[18] that can be performed in a few minutes and results in a semiquantitative measurement of the SCC; however, the test requires a refrigerated sample collected within 5 hours of testing.
- Esterase activity test: A qualitative test that converts the results of an enzymatic reaction into an estimated SCC. Requires 5 to 45 minutes of incubation, depending on the test type.

With regards to cow-side methods, again, not all methods have been researched appropriately. A modified WMT test was evaluated in the laboratory and found to have similar results to electronic somatic cell counting with a high degree of agreement when a threshold of 205,000 cells/mL was used to define an IMI.[18] However,

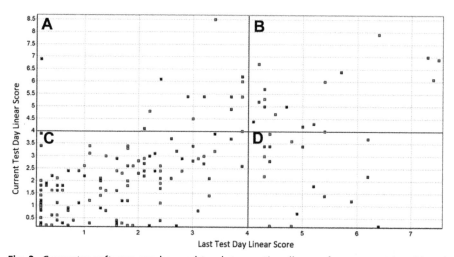

Fig. 2. Computer software can be used to plot somatic cell score from current (y-axis) and previous (x-axis) Dairy Herd Information Association test days to help determine mastitis status. (*A*) Cows with new cases of mastitis (low previous test day somatic cell count [SCC], high current test day SCC). (*B*) Cows with chronic cases of mastitis (high previous test day SCC, high current test day SCC). (*C*) Healthy cows (low previous test day SCC, low current test day SCC). (*D*) Cows with cured cases of mastitis (high previous test day SCC, low current test day SCC). (*Courtesy of* Scott E. Poock, University of Missouri, Columbia, MO.)

when using this same test in a cow-side manner, it markedly underestimated the SCC,[19] making it impractical for on-farm use.

The CMT, when used at a cut point of trace or higher, had a much higher test sensitivity and specificity than the cow-side version of the WMT test. When comparing the CMT, cow-side WMT, and 3 esterase tests, the CMT provided the most accurate, practical, and least cost on-farm screening test to predict subclinical mastitis at dry-off.[20] The CMT also provided a faster and more accurate cow-side screening test to predict subclinical mastitis defined as an SCC of greater than 200,000 cells/mL at dry-off and freshening.[19]

The sensitivity and specificity of the CMT has been evaluated in multiple studies. When evaluating the tests ability to detect an IMI with a major mastitis pathogen (Staphylococcus aureus, Streptococcus spp, and gram-negative organisms) in early lactation, the sensitivity was 82.4% and specificity was 80.6% on day 4 of lactation.[21] When assessed to determine the ability of the CMT to identity IMI with any pathogen, including minor pathogens, the sensitivity was much lower at 61%, but specificity was the same at 80%.[13] When assessing the CMT to identify IMI at dry-off at the cow level for all pathogens, the sensitivity was 70% and specificity was 48%.[22] Overall, although the CMT lacks diagnostic sensitivity for detecting any IMI, when IMI are caused my major pathogens sensitivity is reasonable, suggesting that CMT is still a useful screening tool for the more inflammatory mastitis pathogens.[23]

Other Measures of Mammary Gland Inflammation

Among the other tests available to detect subclinical mastitis discussed at the beginning of this section, few have been validated against reference methods, for example, SCC measurement or detection of IMI, making it challenging to determine which of these is the best detection method. Of those methods that have been evaluated, it has been found that the SCC provides superior diagnostic performance in detecting IMI-negative and IMI-positive cows than LDH and NAGase.[23,24] The milk amyloid A enzyme-linked immunosorbent assay has been shown to be as accurate as the SCC.[25] Other investigators have shown that haptoglobin performs better than milk amyloid A, because a constant increase in the haptoglobin concentration was found in the milk along with increasing quantities of bacterial DNA.[7] Although acute phase proteins may be useful, currently they are not an economically feasible option for diagnosing subclinical mastitis. Like with SCC, cow factors can also affect other measurements used to diagnosis subclinical mastitis, such as LDH and NAGase, and in some cases to a greater extent than SCC.[23]

Although EC is commonly used as an in-line indicator of mastitis, for example, in automated milking systems, its usefulness in detecting cases of mastitis is impacted by multiple factors, including whether the case is clinical or subclinical and changes in milk composition. At the cow-level interquarter comparisons of EC improve test sensitivity and specificity.[26] Hand-held EC meters for cow-side use tend to perform poorly for detecting IMI and seem to be inferior to SCC measurement or CMT. Milk lactose concentration can likewise be measured in-line and has been used to predict IMI.[27] A recent study suggested that, when using attribute weighting analysis of data collected longitudinally during milking (milk volume, protein concentration, lactose concentration, milking time, peak flow, and EC) and comparing these data to 3 SCC thresholds for the detection of subclinical mastitis ($\geq$250,000, $\geq$200,000, or $\geq$150,000 cells/mL), in the absence of SCC, lactose concentration followed by EC were strong indicators of subclinical mastitis.[28]

None of the diagnostic tests used to define mastitis can specify the pathogen causing the infection and, therefore, excludes the information necessary to make a treatment decision. Thus, it is recommended to follow up a diagnosis of mastitis with a diagnostic test to determine the cause of the IMI.

DIAGNOSIS OF INTRAMAMMARY INFECTION

In general, the goals of determining the cause of an IMI are to either select a treatment protocol or determine where control measures need to be implemented or improved on the farm to reduce disease incidence and improve udder health and milk quality. As with SCC, data can be collected at the herd (bulk tank) or pen (in-line sampling), cow, or mammary quarter levels. Bacteriologic culture and polymerase chain reaction (PCR) are the primary methods currently in-use to diagnose IMI. Most PCR assays use real-time multiplex PCR to identify an array of common mastitis pathogens. Regardless of diagnostic method used, there is no true gold standard available to diagnose an IMI.

Culture

Bacterial culture techniques are generally inexpensive and simple to perform, but need to be performed using standardized repeatable methods.[29] Although many mastitis pathogens are readily grown under aerobic conditions on a blood-based agar medium, some pathogens require specific growth media and growth conditions, for example, *Mycoplasma* spp. After culture results are obtained, definitions need to be established to standardize diagnoses.

Standardized methods are described for characterizing bacteria in bulk tank milk.[29] In general, the goals of bulk tank cultures are to (1) monitor raw milk quality and (2) gain herd-level information about the presence of mastitis pathogens, particularly contagious mastitis pathogens such as *S aureus*, *Streptococcus agalactiae*, and *Mycoplasma* spp. The presence of other potential mastitis pathogens in bulk milk may or may not be associated with IMI because many of the other bacteria could come from nonmammary sources, for example, contaminated teat skin and soiled or poorly sanitized milking equipment. The standard plate count (SPC) gives an estimate of the total bacterial load in the bulk tank. The laboratory pasteurized count gives an estimate of thermoduric bacteria (those that survive pasteurization), and the preliminary incubation count estimates the number of psychotropic bacteria (those that grow at cold temperatures). Recommended thresholds for SPC, laboratory pasteurized count, and preliminary incubation count are less than 5000 CFU/mL, less than 100 CFU/mL, and less than 10,000 CFU/mL, respectively.[29] Increases in the SPC, laboratory pasteurized count, and preliminary incubation count can be associated with poor udder cleanliness and/or poor milking system sanitation, but increases in the SPC alone could indicate cases of IMI.

At the cow or mammary quarter level, factors involved in diagnosing an IMI include the number of colonies of the organism isolated from the milk sample, whether the organism is isolated in pure or mixed culture, and if a measure of inflammation is included in the definition. When a quarter milk sample results in the growth of 3 or more colony types, the sample is most likely contaminated.[29] However, it is important to remember that all organisms isolated from a milk sample could be the result of contamination, including known mastitis pathogens such as *S aureus*, *S agalactiae*, and *Mycoplasma* species. Single, duplicate, and triplicate quarter milk samples used in series or in parallel have been used to determined IMI status.

All culture procedures have limited sensitivity and requiring anything other than isolation of 1 colony forming unit (CFU) of an organism from 0.01 mL of milk (100 CFU/ml) further limits the sensitivity.[30] In general, the current recommendation for considering a single quarter sample positive for an IMI is to use 100 CFU/mL, except for non-*aureus Staphylococcus*, where the recommendation is 200 CFU/mL.[30] The use of the results of duplicate and triplicate samples gives high test specificity with a decrease in test sensitivity or results in little gain compared with a single sample.[31] This does not mean the recommended definition stated is always appropriate, because it can depend on the organism isolated, the goals of the farm, and the control program that is planned based on the definition.

Composite milk samples, a sample containing milk from all four quarters of 1 cow, are often used for diagnosis of IMI in cows with subclinical mastitis. In general, composite samples have a low sensitivity, but a high specificity for most organisms.[32] The low sensitivity is caused by the dilution of bacterial numbers by milk from uninfected quarters in the composite sample, similar to the dilution seen with composite SCC. Quarter-level samples are therefore recommended as the first line in mastitis diagnosis, whereas composite samples are useful in surveillance when considering their limitations.[32]

Secondary (Confirmatory) Tests

After primary isolation of a bacterial colony or colonies, additional tests must be applied to determine the identity of the organism. Most laboratories and on-farm culture systems rely on an initial assessment of phenotypic characteristics to help distinguish mastitis pathogens into broad groups. Some common phenotypic tests used to crudely differentiate organisms isolated from milk include visual evaluation of colony morphology, examination of the culture medium for hemolysis, and Gram staining or KOH gelation testing. For gram-positive bacterial isolates, frequently used tests include the catalase test, coagulase test, and CAMP/esculin test to aid in the differentiation of contagious gram-positive bacteria, for example, *S aureus* or *S agalactiae*, from noncontagious gram-positive bacteria, for example, non-*aureus* staphylococci, non-*agalactiae* streptococci, or streptococcal-like organisms. For gram-negative bacterial isolates, growth on selective medium, for example, lactose fermentation on Mac-Conkey agar, as well as triple sugar iron reaction, growth on Simmons citrate agar, oxidase test, and motility testing may be used to differentiate the various environmental gram-negative pathogens. Although these methods are useful for broadly grouping pathogens based on their putative source and also for making preliminary decisions about treatment, they are not entirely accurate.

Historically, further speciation was conducted using proprietary biochemical test panels that, based on colorimetric analysis, yielded a likely bacterial genus and species identity for a given isolate. Available data now suggest that, for some genus and species of bacteria isolated from cases of bovine mastitis, these methods are inaccurate. Hence, other methods to identify organisms to the species level have been explored. Until recently, the most commonly used alternative to biochemical testing was partial sequence analysis of bacterial housekeeping genes, with 16S rRNA being the most universal target.[33] The usefulness of 16S rRNA gene sequencing is limited when applied to certain staphylococcal species owing to the high degree of gene similarity.[34] Therefore, several other housekeeping genes have been used to differentiate staphylococcal species, including, *rpoB*,[35] *tuf*,[36] *sodA*,[37] *gap*,[38] *dnaJ*,[39] and *hsp60*.[40] Although these methods are generally considered accurate, they can be time consuming and costly to perform, and are not always readily available to mastitis diagnostic laboratories.

In the last few years, matrix-assisted laser desorption/ionization time-of-flight (MALDI-TOF) mass spectrometry has been evaluated for the genus and species identification of mastitis pathogens. This technology is becoming widely adopted in many diagnostic and research laboratories. MALDI-TOF is a high-throughput technology that uses a protein fingerprint and a database of reference spectra to determine a bacterial species. This test has been validated as an accurate secondary test for some mastitis pathogens. Overall, MALDI-TOF has been found to be accurate in diagnosis of *Staphylococcus* spp.[41,42] and *Corynebacterium* spp.[43] Although this method has been determined to be a rapid technique for speciation of bacteria, the initial equipment set up is costly and, for the most part, it requires the organism be cultured first. One recent study has determined that MALDI-TOF can be used in a culture-independent fashion to identify bacterial species in experimentally inoculated milk samples. However, the required colony forming unit per milliliter to make an accurate diagnosis was very high, generally much higher than expected in naturally occurring cases of IMI in the field; therefore, direct from milk MALDI-TOF is not currently recommended owing to the high likelihood of false negative results in cows infected with mastitis pathogens.[44]

On-Farm Culture Systems

Although milk cultures can be performed by veterinary practices and diagnostic laboratories, there can be a benefit to having cultures performed on the farm giving producers ready access to timely data for making targeted treatment decisions. On-farm systems can include traditional plating methods using nonselective media such as blood agar or using a combination of selective media such as MacConkey agar for gram-negative pathogens, TKT agar for streptococci, and Baird-Parker for staphylococci.[45] Other simplified options include the use of biplates or triplates that use a combination of these media on a single segregated Petri dish or use of commercially available selective culture films.

Biplate and triplate systems are commercially available. The biplate system has 2 agar types, one for selective growth of gram-negative organisms and one for the selective growth of gram-positive organisms. The triplate has 3 agar types, which in addition to differentiating gram-positive from gram-negative organisms, also helps differentiate staphylococcal species from streptococcal species.[46] Microbial growth films are commercially available for aerobic counts, coliform counts, and staphylococcal counts. One limitation of using the aerobic count bacterial growth film is that it does not allow for species identification, making it impossible to differentiate contamination from an IMI.[47]

With the use of selective medias, it is expected that on-farm culture systems will not detect all mastitis pathogens.[46] These systems are often most successful when interpretation is simplified, such as to differentiate growth from no growth, gram-positive from gram-negative, or for a triplate system, staphylococci from streptococci.[45,46] On-farm culture systems are generally aimed at broadly categorizing mastitis pathogens to select treatment and are not designed to make species-level pathogen diagnoses.[48]

Real-Time Multiplex Polymerase Chain Reaction

Although culture-based methods are still the mainstay in many diagnostic laboratories and veterinary practices for diagnosing IMI, culture-independent methods for identifying bacterial pathogens in milk have become more common over the last decade. The first PCR for the identification of pathogens associated with IMI was made commercially available in 2008. When compared with culture-based methods, PCR is faster, because the results can be provided to the producer within 4 hours, and it has been found to be more sensitive when compared with traditional culture.[49] PCR has been shown to provide a diagnosis for 43% to 47% of mastitic milk samples that were negative based on conventional culture.[50,51] The results of the PCR assay are expressed as a cycle threshold value (Ct); the lower the Ct value, the greater the amount of DNA of the specific pathogen being detected is in the sample and thus the greater the likelihood of a true positive diagnosis. Generally, the cutoff for a positive result is a Ct value of 37.0.[52]

Commercial PCR assays are available for detecting mastitis-causing pathogen DNA in mammary quarter milk samples, cow-level composite milk samples, and bulk tank milk samples. Bulk tank PCR assays can be used in the same way as bulk tank cultures as an indicator of udder health, milking time hygiene, and storage conditions on the farm. Additionally, application of PCR to bulk tank samples can be used to monitor bacteria with low prevalence, such as *S agalactiae*.[53] With that in mind, when using comingled milk (eg, bulk tank or pen) samples, it is recommended to only test for contagious pathogens (such as *S aureus*, *S agalactiae*, and *Mycoplasma* spp.) because there is a high probability that these bacteria originated from the mammary gland.[54]

Commercial PCR tests have been used on cow-level samples collected using an in-line sampling device (such as those used by Dairy Herd Information Association to collect monthly SCC samples). However, it must be remembered that these are not aseptically collected samples and are prone to risk of false-positive results because of teat skin contaminants, contaminated teat orifices, contaminated equipment, and carryover of contaminated milk from other cows.[55,56] Carryover can occur owing to residual milk in the unit, meter, or sampler. Carryover has been found to affect the PCR results for *S aureus* and *S agalactiae* diagnosis. Based on these data, modified cut points have been recommended for *S aureus* diagnosis when using in-line composite samples, with a Ct value of less than 32 being very likely to be infected, a Ct value of greater than 37 very likely to be IMI negative, and a Ct value of 32 to 37 being of undetermined status.[55]

The pros and cons of PCR compared with culture must be acknowledged (**Table 1**). Some concerns with PCR assays include the fact that they only detect the target species that are included in the PCR, which is based on the primer sets included with that

Table 1
Comparison of conventional bacterial culture and PCR-based approaches to diagnosing intramammary infection

	Bacteriologic Culture	PCR
Detects	Bacterial colonies	Bacterial DNA
Diagnostic threshold	CFU/mL	Ct
Live organism	Yes	Not necessarily
Virulence factor detection	Limited (eg, hemolysins)	If PCR primers are included
Factors influencing Se	Growth media and conditions; incubation time; CFU/mL detection threshold/inoculum volume; interpreter	Included primers, primer specificity; Ct threshold
Factors influencing Sp	Contaminated sample; CFU/mL threshold/inoculum volume; interpreter	Contaminated sample; Ct threshold; detection of DNA from nonviable bacteria, primer specificity; carryover when using in-line sampler
Time to result	24 h – 10 d	4 h
Cost	Low	Currently, 4–5 × conventional culture

Abbreviations: CFU, colony forming units; Ct, cycle threshold; PCR, polymerase chain reaction; Se, sensitivity; SP, specificity.

From Middleton JR, Fox LK, Pighetti G, et al. The laboratory handbook on bovine mastitis. Reprinted with permission from the National Mastitis Council Inc., New Prague, Minnesota, USA, 2017. NMC is a not-for-profit organization that provides a forum for the global exchange of information on mastitis control and milk quality. Available at: www.nmconline.org.

specific multiplex kit. There are no guidelines for how to report multispecies results. Additionally, PCR can detect DNA from dead bacteria. In an experimental challenge trail, PCR detected *Staphylococcus* spp. DNA for several days after the bacteria was no longer detected with conventional culture.[57] It is unknown if these were truly dead cells, if the milk contained growth inhibitors preventing bacterial growth on agar, or the bacterial load had dropped below the detection limit of conventional culture, that is, less than 100 CFU/mL.[57] These data are important to consider if PCR is being used as a follow-up test to assess response to treatment. Based on results of Hiitio and co-workers,[57] it is recommend waiting at least 2 to 3 weeks after the onset of mastitis or treatment or until the quarter milk SCC returns to normal levels before using PCR to assess response to treatment.

SUMMARY

The diagnosis of mastitis is generally based on clinical observations or direct or indirect measures of the inflammatory response to infection, whereas the diagnosis of an IMI is based on identification of the infectious agent. Mastitis can be characterized as clinical or subclinical, with subclinical being more common and more challenging to diagnose. SCC or SCS are the most common diagnostic tests used for the detection of subclinical mastitis. Both culture and PCR can be useful in the diagnosis of an IMI; however, both have their advantages and disadvantages. Diagnosing the bacterial agent causing the IMI can help to determine treatment and prevention strategies on the farm, which in turn can help to decrease the incidence and prevalence of mastitis.

REFERENCES

1. Ruegg PL. Managing mastitis and producing quality milk. In: Risco CA, Melendez PR, editors. Dairy production medicine. West Sussex (Shire): John Wiley & Sons; 2011. p. 207–32.
2. Wenz JR, Barrington GM, Garry FB, et al. Use of systemic disease signs to assess disease severity in dairy cows with acute coliform mastitis. J Am Vet Med Assoc 2001;218(4):567–72.
3. Sordillo LM, Shafer-Weaver K, DeRosa D. Immunobiology of the mammary gland. J Dairy Sci 1997;80(8):1851–65.
4. Kitchen BJ. Review of the progress of dairy science: bovine mastitis: milk compositional changes and related diagnostic tests. J Dairy Res 1981;48(1):167–88.
5. Fox LK, Hancock DD, McDonald JS, et al. N-acetyl-beta-D-glucosaminidase activity in whole milk and milk fractions. J Dairy Sci 1988;71(11):2915–22.
6. Kitchen BJ, Middleton G, Salmon M. Bovine milk N-acetyl-beta-D-glucosaminidase and its significance in the detection of abnormal udder secretions. J Dairy Res 1978;45(1):15–20.
7. Kalmus P, Simojoki H, Pyorala S, et al. Milk haptoglobin, milk amyloid A, and N-acetyl-beta-D-glucosaminidase activity in bovines with naturally occurring clinical mastitis diagnosed with a quantitative PCR test. J Dairy Sci 2013;96(6):3662–70.
8. McDermott MP, Erb HN, Natzke RP. Predictability by somatic cell counts related to prevalence of intrammary infection within herds. J Dairy Sci 1982;65(8):1535–9.
9. Reksen O, Solverod L, Osteras O. Relationships between milk culture results and composite milk somatic cell counts in Norwegian dairy cattle. J Dairy Sci 2008;91(8):3102–13.
10. Jashari R, Piepers S, De Vliegher S. Evaluation of the composite milk somatic cell count as a predictor of intramammary infection in dairy cattle. J Dairy Sci 2016;99(11):9271–86.

11. Schukken YH, Wilson DJ, Welcome F, et al. Monitoring udder health and milk quality using somatic cell counts. Vet Res 2003;34(5):579–96.
12. Djabri B, Bareille N, Beaudeau F, et al. Quarter milk somatic cell count in infected dairy cows: a meta-analysis. Vet Res 2002;33(4):335–57.
13. Middleton JR, Hardin D, Steevens B, et al. Use of somatic cell counts and California mastitis test results from individual quarter milk samples to detect subclinical intramammary infection in dairy cattle from a herd with a high bulk tank somatic cell count. J Am Vet Med Assoc 2004;224(3):419–23.
14. Schepers AJ, Lam TJ, Schukken YH, et al. Estimation of variance components for somatic cell counts to determine thresholds for uninfected quarters. J Dairy Sci 1997;80(8):1833–40.
15. Brolund L. Cell counts in bovine milk. Causes of variation and applicability for diagnosis of subclinical mastitis. Acta Vet Scand Suppl 1985;80:1–123.
16. Harmon RJ. Physiology of mastitis and factors affecting somatic cell counts. J Dairy Sci 1994;77(7):2103–12.
17. Walsh S, Buckley F, Berry DP, et al. Effects of breed, feeding system, and parity on udder health and milking characteristics. J Dairy Sci 2007;90(12):5767–79.
18. Rodrigues AC, Cassoli LD, Machado PF, et al. Short communication: evaluation of an on-farm test to estimate somatic cell count. J Dairy Sci 2009;92(3):990–5.
19. Kandeel SA, Megahed AA, Arnaout FK, et al. Evaluation and comparison of 2 on-farm tests for estimating somatic cell count in quarter milk samples from lactating dairy cattle. J Vet Intern Med 2018;32(1):506–15.
20. Kandeel SA, Megahed AA, Constable PD. Comparison of six on-farm tests to estimate somatic cell count at dry-off in dairy cattle. Paper presented at: American College of Veterinary Internal Medicine Forum 2017. National Harbor, MD, June 8-9, 2017. p.1358.
21. Dingwell RT, Leslie KE, Schukken YH, et al. Evaluation of the California mastitis test to detect an intramammary infection with a major pathogen in early lactation dairy cows. Can Vet J 2003;44(5):413–5.
22. Sanford CJ, Keefe GP, Sanchez J, et al. Test characteristics from latent-class models of the California Mastitis Test. Prev Vet Med 2006;77(1–2):96–108.
23. Nyman AK, Persson Waller K, Bennedsgaard TW, et al. Associations of udder-health indicators with cow factors and with intramammary infection in dairy cows. J Dairy Sci 2014;97(9):5459–73.
24. Nyman AK, Emanuelson U, Waller KP. Diagnostic test performance of somatic cell count, lactate dehydrogenase, and N-acetyl-beta-D-glucosaminidase for detecting dairy cows with intramammary infection. J Dairy Sci 2016;99(2):1440–8.
25. Jaeger S, Virchow F, Torgerson PR, et al. Test characteristics of milk amyloid A ELISA, somatic cell count, and bacteriological culture for detection of intramammary pathogens that cause subclinical mastitis. J Dairy Sci 2017;100(9):7419–26.
26. Jensen NE, Knudsen K. Interquarter comparison of markers of subclinical mastitis: somatic cell count, electrical conductivity, N-acetyl-beta-glucosaminidase and antitrypsin. J Dairy Res 1991;58(4):389–99.
27. Pyorala S. Indicators of inflammation in the diagnosis of mastitis. Vet Res 2003;34(5):565–78.
28. Ebrahimie E, Ebrahimi F, Ebrahimi M, et al. A large-scale study of indicators of sub-clinical mastitis in dairy cattle by attribute weighting analysis of milk composition features: highlighting the predictive power of lactose and electrical conductivity. J Dairy Res 2018;85(2):193–200.
29. Middleton JR, Fox LK, Pighetti G, et al. Laboratory handbook on bovine mastitis. New Prague (MN): National Mastitis Council; 2017.

30. Dohoo IR, Smith J, Andersen S, et al. Diagnosing intramammary infections: evaluation of definitions based on a single milk sample. J Dairy Sci 2011;94(1):250–61.

31. Dohoo I, Andersen S, Dingwell R, et al. Diagnosing intramammary infections: comparison of multiple versus single quarter milk samples for the identification of intramammary infections in lactating dairy cows. J Dairy Sci 2011;94(11): 5515–22.

32. Reyher KK, Dohoo IR. Diagnosing intramammary infections: evaluation of composite milk samples to detect intramammary infections. J Dairy Sci 2011;94(7):3387–96.

33. Patel JB. 16S rRNA gene sequencing for bacterial pathogen identification in the clinical laboratory. Mol Diagn 2001;6(4):313–21.

34. Becker K, Harmsen D, Mellmann A, et al. Development and evaluation of a quality-controlled ribosomal sequence database for 16S ribosomal DNA-based identification of *Staphylococcus* species. J Clin Microbiol 2004;42(11):4988–95.

35. Drancourt M, Raoult D. *rpoB* gene sequence-based identification of *Staphylococcus* species. J Clin Microbiol 2002;40(4):1333–8.

36. Hwang SM, Kim MS, Park KU, et al. Tuf gene sequence analysis has greater discriminatory power than 16S rRNA sequence analysis in identification of clinical isolates of coagulase-negative staphylococci. J Clin Microbiol 2011;49(12): 4142–9.

37. Poyart C, Quesne G, Boumaila C, et al. Rapid and accurate species-level identification of coagulase-negative staphylococci by using the *sodA* gene as a target. J Clin Microbiol 2001;39(12):4296–301.

38. Ghebremedhin B, Layer F, Konig W, et al. Genetic classification and distinguishing of *Staphylococcus* species based on different partial gap, 16S rRNA, *hsp60*, *rpoB*, *sodA*, and *tuf* gene sequences. J Clin Microbiol 2008;46(3):1019–25.

39. Shah MM, Iihara H, Noda M, et al. *dnaJ* gene sequence-based assay for species identification and phylogenetic grouping in the genus *Staphylococcus*. Int J Syst Evol Microbiol 2007;57(Pt 1):25–30.

40. Kwok AY, Su SC, Reynolds RP, et al. Species identification and phylogenetic relationships based on partial HSP60 gene sequences within the genus *Staphylococcus*. Int J Syst Bacteriol 1999;49(Pt 3):1181–92.

41. Cameron M, Barkema HW, De Buck J, et al. Identification of bovine-associated coagulase-negative staphylococci by matrix-assisted laser desorption/ionization time-of-flight mass spectrometry using a direct transfer protocol. J Dairy Sci 2017;100(3):2137–47.

42. Cameron M, Perry J, Middleton JR, et al. Short communication: evaluation of MALDI-TOF mass spectrometry and a custom reference spectra expanded database for the identification of bovine-associated coagulase-negative staphylococci. J Dairy Sci 2018;101(1):590–5.

43. Goncalves JL, Tomazi T, Barreiro JR, et al. Identification of *Corynebacterium* spp. isolated from bovine intramammary infections by matrix-assisted laser desorption ionization-time of flight mass spectrometry. Vet Microbiol 2014;173(1–2):147–51.

44. Barreiro JR, Goncalves JL, Braga PAC, et al. Non-culture-based identification of mastitis-causing bacteria by MALDI-TOF mass spectrometry. J Dairy Sci 2017; 100(4):2928–34.

45. Ruegg PL. On-farm diagnosis of mastitis infections and organisms. Paper presented at: National Mastitis Council Regional Meeting 2005. Burlington, VT, July 12-13, 2005. p. 24-30.

46. Godden S, Lago A, Bey R, et al. Dingwell. Use of on-farm culture systems in mastitis control programs. Paper presented at: National Mastitis Council Regional Meeting 2007. Visalia, CA, May 22-23, 2007. p. 1–9.

47. Cameron M, Keefe GP, Roy JP, et al. Evaluation of a 3M Petrifilm on-farm culture system for the detection of intramammary infection at the end of lactation. Prev Vet Med 2013;111(1–2):1–9.
48. Royster E, Godden S, Goulart D, et al. Evaluation of the Minnesota Easy Culture System II Bi-Plate and Tri-Plate for identification of common mastitis pathogens in milk. J Dairy Sci 2014;97(6):3648–59.
49. Koskinen MT, Wellenberg GJ, Sampimon OC, et al. Field comparison of real-time polymerase chain reaction and bacterial culture for identification of bovine mastitis bacteria. J Dairy Sci 2010;93(12):5707–15.
50. Taponen S, Salmikivi L, Simojoki H, et al. Real-time polymerase chain reaction-based identification of bacteria in milk samples from bovine clinical mastitis with no growth in conventional culturing. J Dairy Sci 2009;92(6):2610–7.
51. Bexiga R, Koskinen MT, Holopainen J, et al. Diagnosis of intramammary infection in samples yielding negative results or minor pathogens in conventional bacterial culturing. J Dairy Res 2011;78(1):49–55.
52. Koskinen MT, Holopainen J, Pyorala S, et al. Analytical specificity and sensitivity of a real-time polymerase chain reaction assay for identification of bovine mastitis pathogens. J Dairy Sci 2009;92(3):952–9.
53. Katholm J, Bennedsgaard TW, Koskinen MT, et al. Quality of bulk tank milk samples from Danish dairy herds based on real-time polymerase chain reaction identification of mastitis pathogens. J Dairy Sci 2012;95(10):5702–8.
54. Kelton DF, Godkin MA. Frequently asked questions about the Pathoproof mastitis 3 PCR assay. Paper presented at: NMC 53rd Annual Meeting 2014. Fort Worth, TX, January 26-28, 2014. p. 127–32.
55. Mahmmod YS, Klaas IC, Enevoldsen C. DNA carryover in milk samples from routine milk recording used for PCR-based diagnosis of bovine *Staphylococcus aureus* mastitis. J Dairy Sci 2017;100(7):5709–16.
56. Mahmmod YS, Mweu MM, Nielsen SS, et al. Effect of carryover and presampling procedures on the results of real-time PCR used for diagnosis of bovine intramammary infections with *Streptococcus agalactiae* at routine milk recordings. Prev Vet Med 2014;113(4):512–21.
57. Hiitio H, Simojoki H, Kalmus P, et al. The effect of sampling technique on PCR-based bacteriological results of bovine milk samples. J Dairy Sci 2016; 99(8):6532–41.

Optimization of Clinical Mastitis Records on Dairies

John R. Wenz, DVM, MS

KEYWORDS

- Clinical mastitis • Records • Data management

KEY POINTS

- Deriving value from clinical mastitis (CM) records requires accurate and consistent records and the tools for their efficient summary and analysis.
- Variation in CM case definition or detection intensity across dairies does not preclude consistent data recording on each dairy.
- Dairy management software can improve consistency of CM records by prompting users for quarter(s) affected, treatment, and severity at minimum.
- User-defined record systems must establish and follow protocols for CM data recording. All records must have the same information in the same order and use the same abbreviations to allow efficient summary and analysis of udder health management by computer applications.
- CM episodes should be recorded at the quarter level. Cow-level recording compromises record consistency and accuracy of outcomes assessed, such as recurrence when multiple quarters are concurrently affected.

INTRODUCTION

The value of clinical mastitis (CM) records to monitor and thus effectively manage udder health is well known. Or is it? If it is so valuable, why has there not been industry-wide adoption of CM recording standards as exist for milk production? Why is CM data entry not controlled in the most common dairy management software (DMS) to ensure consistent records? Why does DMS not provide features that enable the efficient summary and analysis of CM records like they do for reproduction data? Why are most dairy producers not routinely using commonly recommended udder health key performance indicators (KPIs) besides somatic cell count (SCC)? The simple answer is a real or perceived lack of value among players in the industry.

In reference to farm financial records, Hardaker and Anderson[1] suggested the lack of adoption of recording systems was likely associated with a failure to meet the needs

Conflicts: The author has financial interest in a company that licensed the HEALTHSUM technology from Washington State University.
Field Disease Investigation Unit, Department of Clinical Sciences, College of Veterinary Medicine, Washington State University, PO Box 646610, Pullman, WA 99164-6610, USA
E-mail address: jrwenz@wsu.edu

of a majority of users. Perhaps dairies do not need the ability to routinely analyze CM KPIs. More likely it is a latent need or one that is not realized due to a lack of knowledge or availability of a ready solution. Many dairy herds have effectively controlled contagious mastitis pathogens through standard mastitis control plans and focusing on SCC analysis. The industry continues to rely on those same actions to address CM due to environmental mastitis pathogens. They are not, however, proving as effective as it seems they once were. The risks factors for environmental pathogens are different and arguably more complex. Previously, the battles were limited to milking time or the parlor; now they are waged all the time almost everywhere on the dairy. Milking machines, parlors, and their challenges varied but not to the extent seen in the environment of cows across the industry. Better intelligence is needed to access the effectiveness of udder health management plans to combat environmental pathogens. This requires reliable data from the field and the tools to derive knowledge from those data.

Etherington and colleagues,[2] in a review of dairy data management identified a "Lack of uniformity with respect to data entry" as a disadvantage of on-farm data recording systems and suggested this problem could be overcome with "the design of prospective standardized data recording and entry conventions." In a review of general requirements for health data, Kelton and colleagues[3] stated, "The most complete, accurate and consistent data is worthless if it is not accessible in a form that allows data to be aggregated and analyzed." Despite a long-standing recognition of these problems, CM data are not uniform and the tools to efficiently analyze those data to generate actionable knowledge are limited. Each of these factors is both a cause and effect. The situation can be viewed as a cycle (**Fig. 1**). This cycle can be a virtuous one with favorable results but likely requires effort at 2 critical points: data entry as well as summary and analysis to start and maintain a positive cycle. Until data entry is controlled by DMS, standard CM recording protocols need to be implemented to ensure accurate, consistent (ie, computer-friendly) data are available. Increased time commitment is a common concern when implementing standard health data recording protocols. A study of 22 dairies, however, showed no change or a reduction in time required for data capture (96% of dairies) and data entry (77% of dairies).[4] Those dairies with increased data entry time were not recording health data in the computer before the study.

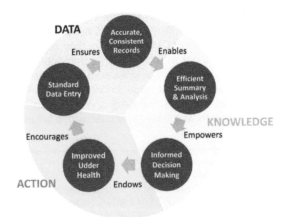

Fig. 1. CM data value cycle illustrating the steps involved in creating value as data produce knowledge resulting in action reinforcing the value of data quality. Standard data entry and efficient summary and analysis are both critical to start and maintain the cycle.

The full value of CM data cannot be realized until applications to efficiently summarize and analyze those data are widely available. Such tools will allow a better understanding of CM on individual dairies and benchmarking. Benchmarking involves measurement and reporting of KPIs and comparison with peers. Studies have shown benchmarking improved management of dairy cattle lameness, calf growth, and passive transfer of immunity.[5–7] Furthermore, it can facilitate a more data-driven approach to management and provide evidence of the value of data recording efforts (see **Fig. 1**).

Disparate disease definitions are a common concern about the validity of benchmarking across dairies. Different disease definitions do not preclude the accurate and consistent recording of CM as defined on each dairy. Benchmarking can motivate farmers through pride in performance and better knowledge of their operation in the context of others.[7] Awareness of how differences in disease definition and recording practices can diminish the value of benchmarking may provide the motivation to adopt standard practices. This article focuses on considerations to optimize CM data recording and analysis that should improve udder health management.

ASSESSING UDDER HEALTH MANAGEMENT

KPIs are those metrics that answer the questions people need to know to do their jobs effectively to meet the objectives of the business. There are both lagging and leading indicators. Lagging indicators are outputs that generally are easily measured but have multiple inputs, thus can be harder to change, and there is usually a time delay before the change is observed. Leading indicators focus on those inputs that can be more easily changed but are often harder or take additional effort to measure. Both are needed to inform people how well they have done and are doing their job. Total quality management principles focus on monitoring and controlling variation in the inputs to ensure a consistently high-quality output. Yet leading indicators are typically evaluated for only a limited time as a reaction to a defect in the output (eg, investigation of an excessively high incidence of CM). This approach is flawed for several reasons. One, it is too late; the defect in udder health has already occurred. Two, evaluation of the inputs (eg, bedding and cow hygiene, coverage of predip) for a short time (often only 1 point in time) may fail to identify variation that lead to the problem. Three, failure to continue monitoring the inputs means future variations that will have a negative impact on udder health will go undetected and quality defects will occur again and again. The last point is not true for some herds with the managerial capability to facilitate the consistent, effective implementation of intended best management practices by their people (ie, have a consistently low CM incidence and bulk tank SCC). Yet, most herds would benefit from routine monitoring of these leading indicators. In many cases, however, adding monitoring activities to an already overburdened management team is unwise. This presents opportunity for veterinarians to deliver value to clients by providing a needed service.

The overarching questions that address the strategic objectives of udder health management are (1) Is the management plan to prevent intramammary infections consistently effective? and (2) When infections occur, does the therapeutic plan efficiently eliminate them? Numerous udder health KPIs addressing both subclinical and clinical infections have been described well in the literature.[8–13] Readers are referred to the previous literature for details on their calculation and interpretation. The focus of this article is on how CM data should be recorded so those KPI can be effectively monitored. Indicators assessing the impact of the dry period on CM incidence and the outcomes of CM episodes are highlighted.

ACHIEVING ACCURATE AND CONSISTENT CLINICAL MASTITIS RECORDS

Until DMS provides system control of data entry, free-form entry needs to be governed by standard protocols on each dairy. Veterinarians are positioned well to deliver value to their dairy clients by facilitating data management protocol development and implementation. The capture of needed data should be integrated into CM identification and treatment protocols and, in some cases, is entered directly into the computer system with a remote device. Data capture typically happens, however, through written records that are later entered into the computer. When data are manually entered into the computer specific data entry protocols are needed. Detailed protocol setup guides to achieve good health records are available at www.goodhealthrecords.com. The 3 simple rules of good recording (**Box 1**) highlight the key recommendations guiding protocols for CM data recording. What follows is a description of those recommendations and recording practices that commonly compromise CM record quality.

Record All Clinical Mastitis Episodes at the Quarter Level

For CM records to be an accurate reflection of true disease in the herd, all cases that are identified must be recorded. Often the motivation to keep CM records is based on management of the individual cow and avoidance of antibiotic residues. Thus, the focus is on recording treatments and it is logical that clinical episodes not treated may not get recorded. Everyone involved in the process needs to share the same goals of recording and understand the objectives. When the goal of recording is to monitor udder health management at the individual level and herd level, with the objectives of assessing prevention and therapeutic efficacy, the value of recording all CM episodes regardless of treatment or severity is more apparent.

Common reasons CM episodes are not recorded (**Box 2**) should be specifically addressed in CM data recording protocols and routinely monitored. Failure to record CM episodes that were not treated often are identified by routine comparison of hospital written records and mastitis events recorded in the computer. Consistent removal of cows without recording a CM episodes can be identified by generating a list of cows sold or died with a reason of mastitis recorded and spot checking individual cow records for a related CM event. Failure to record a CM episode for cows where the decision was to stop milking the quarter can similarly be identified by generating a list of cows with an event denoting that decision (eg, 3TEAT). None should be found but, if it is, those cows should also have a CM event recorded (see **Box 2**).

CM episodes cannot be recorded if they are not identified. Detection intensity is the proportion of IMI exhibiting clinical signs that are identified.[9] Detection intensity is influenced by the observational skill of milkers, which is a function of training, motivation, and employee turnover. Ruegg[9] recommends using the severity distribution of

---

Box 1
Three simple rules of good recording to ensure accurate, consistent clinical mastitis records

1. Record all CM episodes at the quarter level.

2. Use a single, specific event (eg, MAST). Use different events to record retreatments (eg, REMAST) and daily treatments (eg, DLYMAST) of a CM episode or treatment of cows with high SCC (eg, HISCC).

3. Record consistent event remarks that
   a. Contain the same information (eg, treatment, quarter, culture, and severity)
   b. Are in the same order
   c. Use the same abbreviations (eg, NT [no treatment])

Box 2
Common reasons clinical mastitis episodes do not get recorded

- No antimicrobial treatment was given. No treatment is a therapeutic decision. The episode should still be recorded with "no treatment" as the treatment. Always differentiate between a "no treat" with the intent of keeping the cow (eg, NT) and one where the intent is to immediately sell the cow (eg, BF [beef]). This is important when evaluating removal as an outcome of a decision not to treat where those not treated because they were to be sold should not be included.

- The cow was sold or died, and mastitis was recorded as the reason. It is good to record consistent removal reasons; however, the CM episode should still be recorded as a disease event.

- Decision to stop milking the quarter. Often this is recorded as a separate event (eg, 3TEAT). This is a treatment decision, however, and should be recorded as a treatment within a CM record for that episode.

- Cow-level recording of CM. When multiple quarters are affected during the same CM episode, limited space to record data can result in loss of quarter episode information.

CM cases to assess detection intensity. Inadequate detection of severity score 1, or mild, cases should be suspected when greater than 20% of CM cases are a severity score 3, or severe.

Use a Single, Specific Event to Record Clinical Mastitis Episodes

CM episodes should be recorded using a single, specific event (eg, MAST) to provide an accurate count of CM incidence. Common situations where a different event should be recorded (**Box 3**) should be specifically addressed in CM data recording protocols to avoid inflation of CM incidence. When all the information about a CM episode does not fit in the space available, multiple CM episode events may be recorded to capture the desired information. This typically occurs with severe CM episodes receiving supportive care. Recommended best practice is to establish a treatment abbreviation that represents all the treatments given. Alternatively, record quarter and intramammary treatment using the CM event (eg, MAST) and supportive care treatments in a different event (eg, MASTX). A high apparent incidence of CM in all 4 quarters of the same cow of approximately 7 to 10 days in milk is suggestive of improper recording of cows treated for a positive, composite fresh milk culture and should be investigated. Improper recording of cows with high SCC being treated should be investigated when a spike in CM episodes recorded on the same day is observed shortly after a test date.

Box 3
Situations where a different event from the one used to record clinical mastitis episodes (eg, MAST) should be recorded to avoid inflation of clinical mastitis incidence

- Retreatment of a CM episode in the same quarter (eg, use REMAST)
- Daily treatments of a CM episode (eg, use DLYMAST)
- Cows treated for high SCC (eg, use HISCC) or a positive fresh cow milk culture (eg, use FMAST)
- Cows with blood in otherwise normal milk (eg, use BLOOD)
- Recording multiple MAST events to capture all information about a CM episode (eg, use MASTX)

Record Consistent Event Remarks

Consistency is critical for computer-friendly records that can be efficiently summarized and analyzed and provide the knowledge needed to effectively manage udder health. Protocols for CM records should specify the information that will be recorded for all CM cases. At minimum, the quarter and treatment should be recorded to evaluate outcomes of a CM episode. Consistent abbreviations should be used. Two-character abbreviations are recommended because they are the easiest to interpret while maximizing the information recorded when space is limited. Finally, each record should have the information in the same order so it can be parsed out by software applications. An example is treatment as 2 characters (TX), followed by quarter as 2 characters (QQ) (eg, TXQQ). If the character number of abbreviations is variable, then that information should come at the end of the remark, where it does not disrupt the expected character number and order of the information or be separated by a delimiter (**Fig. 2**).

Common data entry errors (**Box 4**) leading to inconsistent CM records should be specifically addressed in CM data recording protocols to avoid loss of data and keep records computer friendly. As discussed previously, when record keeping is focused on data on all CM episodes and their management rather than solely treatments, quality is improved. When the focus is on recording treatments, when no treatment is given, there is no perceived need to record treatment and often quarter is not recorded either. Such data entry errors can simply be evaluated by generating a list of cows with a CM event and scanning for those missing quarter or treatment information. Quarter affected should always be recorded so the outcomes of the CM episode can be evaluated. As described in **Box 3**, no treatment is a therapeutic decision and should be recorded in a way that differentiates between episodes not treated with the intent of keeping the cow versus immediate removal. If information about a CM episode is not known, a placeholder abbreviation should be use to maintain the expected order of the information. For example, if a 2-character abbreviation is used for treatment TX could be used when that information is not known.

Functions within DMS should be used to foster consistency of CM records. Default event remarks can be set using the Protocols function of DairyComp 305 (VAS, Tulare, California). Entries into the HthDiag field of DHI-Plus (Amelicor, Provo, Utah) can be

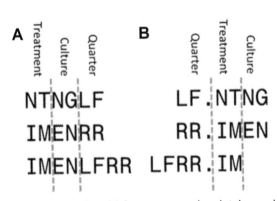

Fig. 2. Alternative ways to record multiple quarters and maintain consistency that allow data parsing by computer. (*A*) Quarter with variable character number at end. (*B*) Use of delimiter (*dot*) to separate variable and consistent character number abbreviations. Dashed vertical lines denote where the data are parsed. Fixed width parsing can be accomplished when the variable character information comes at the end.

Box 4
Data entry errors leading to inconsistent clinical mastitis records

- Information is not recorded
  - Most common is quarter ± treatment of CM episode not treated with an intramammary antibiotic
- Information is recorded using variable character number abbreviations
  - Most common is a CM episode with multiple affected quarters entered as a single CM record
- Variation in the digits recorded for a number
  - Most common is pen number cow was in when detected (eg, 3 and 10 should be 03 and 10)
- Extraneous information not specified in protocol is recorded
  - For example, COLI, MYCO, STAUR, SICK, BEEF, CULL, and SELL

---

standardized by defining macros. Although these functions are available, many herds may not be implementing them to improve data quality. Only 42% of 50 herds using DairyComp 305 used the protocols function.[14] Lack of knowledge of how these functions work may be a reason they are not used. Details on their use to improve the consistency of health records can be found at www.goodhealthrecords.com.

Record Clinical Mastitis at the Quarter Level

CM should be recorded and evaluated at the quarter level. Most herds keeping CM records are likely already recording quarter. A study of 50 large herds using Dairy-Comp 305 found that of the 42 recording CM, 86% recorded the quarter affected whereas only 67% recorded treatment.[14]

Management of CM is most commonly performed at the quarter level, ideally guided by milk culture results. Consider a cow with 2 quarters affected (left front [LF] and right rear [RR]), one that yields no growth (NG) and the other an environmental streptococci (EN). The mastitis treatment protocol for the first CM episode of a lactation is NT of NG and an intramammary antibiotic (IM) of EN. It is clear from this example that a separate record of the affected quarters is necessary to accurately capture all the information about CM case management in free-form systems with limited space. Even if culture results are not available, outcomes should be evaluated at the quarter level (discussed later).

In the previous example, the information to be recorded was treatment, culture result, and quarter: NTNGLF and IMENRR. When recorded at the cow level, information is lost if space is limited and typically what is omitted is that which did not result in drug administration (the NT of the NG in the LF quarter). The CM record is then not accurate and outcomes of the omitted no growth quarter episode cannot be assessed. When there is resistance to recording each quarter as a separate event, accuracy of the records is lost but consistency of CM records can be preserved in 1 of 3 ways. The first is to record quarter information last if the abbreviations are variable in length (eg, LF and LFRF, 2 and 4 characters). The data can still be parsed out by a computer (see **Fig. 2**A). The second is to use a delimiter, such as a period (.) or slash (/), to separate the data (see **Fig. 2**B). This allows a computer to parse out a variable length abbreviation (like quarter, in this example) and then parse the remaining data by character number. The third way is to record all possible quarter combinations with a 2-character abbreviation (**Table 1**).

Accurate assessment of the outcomes of CM cases requires quarter-level recording. Retreatment needs to be evaluated at the quarter level. Recurrent clinical episodes in the same quarter may be associated with failure of treatment to

Table 1
Two-character abbreviations for all possible multiple-quarter combinations

Quarters	Abbreviation
LF LR RF RR	AL
LF LR	BL or LS
RF RR	BR or RS
LF RF	BF
LR RR	BH
LF RR	LX
RF LR	RX
3 Quarters	Reverse letters of unaffected quarter using HR for RR

Abbreviations: AL, all; BL, both left; LS, left side; BR, both right; RS, right side; BF, both front; BH both hind. LX and RX are defined by the Quarters they represent.

achieve a bacteriologic cure or failure to prevent a new IMI that results in CM. By contrast, a subsequent episode in a different quarter likely represents a prevention failure in herds that have successfully controlled contagious pathogens.

EVALUATING OUTCOMES OF CLINICAL MASTITIS EPISODES

Udder health monitoring should, at minimum, allow routine assessment of the prevention and therapeutic plan efficacy on a dairy. The incidence of CM is a measure of prevention efficacy; however, it can also be influenced by the therapeutic management of clinical cases. Five KPIs that assess the outcomes of CM episodes are considered (**Box 5**). Switch treatment and retreatment are primarily focused on antibiotic treatments and their effectiveness. Recurrence and lost quarter can be influenced by both prevention and treatment failures whereas removal can be seen as the ultimate failure of udder health management. Calculation of these metrics requires specific data, thus determining the CM recording protocol for a dairy. An objective of the protocol is to provide the most accurate record of the management of each CM episode of a cow at the quarter-level. This is facilitated by recording retreatments using a different event (eg, REMAST) than the one used to record a new CM episode (eg, MAST). Regardless of the events used, for consistency in the industry, definition of a retreatment versus a recurrence in the same quarter should be defined based on the days between 2 recorded CM episodes. Fourteen days is commonly used to define CM episodes.[15–20] This cutpoint was based on the average duration of CM caused by environmental mastitis pathogens.[21]

Box 5
Key performance indicators to assess management of clinical mastitis

- SWITCH—switch treatment before initial course is completed.
- RETREAT - Retreatment: administration of a second course of treatment after the first is complete
- RECUR - Recurrence: subsequent CM episode in the same quarter greater than 14 days after the first
- LOSTQ - Lost quarter: decision is made to stop milking the quarter. Should be recorded as a treatment of a CM episode
- REMOVE—cows SOLD or DIED within a specified number of days of a CM episode

Switch Treatment

Switch treatment is primarily a measure of treatment protocol compliance where there is a switch in intramammary antibiotics before the initial course of treatment is completed. It could also reflect a valid protocol change due to increased severity. Protocol noncompliance is identified when the days between recorded episodes in the same quarter are fewer than the expected duration of treatment, the treatment is different, and there is no indication of a change in severity. Evaluating switch treatments requires recording of treatment, treatment duration, quarter, and severity.

Retreatment

Retreatment of CM episodes is a measure of the effectiveness of initial treatment focused on intramammary antibiotics. When retreatment is recorded using a different event than the one used to record a new CM episode (eg, REMAST), it can be defined as the administration of a second treatment protocol after the first is complete. The days between the initial CM episode and the retreatment (REMAST) event in the same quarter would be greater than the expected duration of treatment but less than or equal to 14 days. When a different event is not used, retreatment is defined as a subsequent episode recorded greater than the expected days of treatment but less than or equal to 14 days with the same or different treatment. Evaluation of retreatment requires recording of treatment, duration of treatment, and quarter.

Defining retreatment is difficult in herds that treat for a variable number of days based on clinical assessment. One method is to determine the average days of treatment of each CM episode during a defined time period and consider any episode with a days treated greater than the average to be retreated. Evaluating the distribution of treatment days also may be informative. Many herds that treat for a variable number of days record each day of treatment. Recording daily treatments as a separate event (eg, DLYMAST) facilitates enumeration of days treated and avoids inflation of CM incidence.

Recurrence

Recurrence is best defined as a subsequent CM episode in the same quarter recorded greater than 14 days after the first (or after the last retreatment episode of the first). It can be influenced by initial treatment efficacy and prevention efficacy. Comparison of milk culture results, when available, can facilitate interpretation. Recognizing the limitations (sensitivity) of aerobic milk culture, those results can be useful. Different bacterial isolates is good evidence of a new IMI and prevention failure, whereas the same bacterial isolate from both episodes may be more a reflection of therapeutic failure. It has been shown that the risk of recurrence is increased when bacteriologic cure is not achieved.[16,22] When infection pressure is high, however, a greater proportion of recurrent CM episodes may be due to new IMI after bacteriologic cure of a previous infection.

A study in New Zealand of 27 recurrent CM episodes due to *Stretococcus uberis*, where strain was determined by pulse-field gel electrophoresis, found a majority (74%) were caused by a new strain rather than a persistent strain.[23] A conclusion of the study was that treatment failure may not be a common reason for recurrence, and cow and environmental exposure factors were more important. Recurrent episodes, however, were defined at the cow level, not quarter level. Of the 20 episodes with a different strain, 16 (80%) were episodes in a different quarter. Evaluating the strains obtained from the same quarters would provide a better understanding of the role of treatment failure in recurrence. A Brazilian study investigated risk factors for 2 successive cases of CM in the same lactation in 113 cows compared with 324 control cows that only had 1 CM episode.[20] In that study of 2 herds, a recurrent case was also defined at the cow level rather than quarter level, and 51% (58 cows) had the subsequent case in a different quarter. Of the 55 cows that recurred in the same quarter, 29% had identical milk culture results from both episodes and only 1 cow was infected with *Staphylococcus aureus*. The isolates from different quarter cases was not reported. Although contagious pathogens were considered controlled in the study herds, the average bulk tank SCCs reported were 346,000 cells/mL and 366,000 cells/mL for herds A and B, respectively. Of the cows enrolled from herd A, 4 and 1 had an episode where *Staphylococcus aureus* and *Streptococcus agalactiae* were isolated, respectively. No contagious pathogens were isolated from herd B. A majority of cases were associated with environmental pathogens. Together with the relatively high bulk tank SCC, this suggests a high environmental infection pressure and may explain why only 29% of same quarter recurrent episodes had the same milk culture result. This is important to consider because the investigators suggest these results along with those of Abureema and colleagues[23] support teat and udder characteristics as more important factors for recurrence than therapeutic failure. Interpretation of same quarter recurrence in the context of the first case incidence rate may be informative.

For the purpose of monitoring udder health management on a dairy, an end point for days to recurrence is needed to define a consistent risk period for evaluation. The longer the defined risk period, the greater lag in obtaining the value and time for a recurrence to occur. It is recommended that the days to recurrence be calculated for all such episodes and then analysis can be limited to the risk period of interest. The cumulative percentage of recurrent clinical episodes (n = 7972) in the same quarter by days to recurrence on 5 Holstein dairies in the Western United States was evaluated (**Fig. 3**) (John R. Wenz, DVM, MS, unpublished data, 2018). It is interesting to note the variation between herds, in particular herd B, that had a substantially lower rate of recurrence primarily by 30 days. This could reflect a better overall

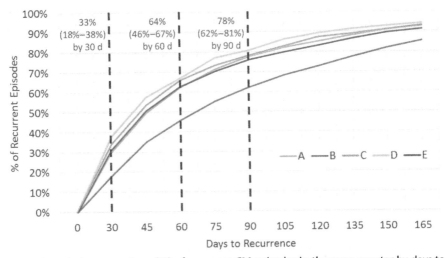

Fig. 3. Cumulative percentage (%) of recurrent CM episodes in the same quarter by days to recurrence for 5 Holstein dairies (A–E) in the Western United States. Data represent 7972 recurrent episodes. The minimum days to recurrence was 15 days and the maximum days to recurrence was 478 days.

therapeutic outcome in that herd. Further work evaluating the epidemiology of recurrent CM episodes, including days to recurrence, culture result, treatment, and first case incidence rate, is needed. Evaluation of recurrence requires recording of quarter at minimum. Culture result is desirable to help differentiate recurrence due to therapeutic versus prevention failure.

Lost Quarter

Lost quarter, often recorded as 3TEAT, is both an outcome and a treatment of CM where the decision is made to stop milking that quarter. Most lost quarters are the result of multiple CM recurrent episodes or a single episode refractory to treatment. It should be recorded as the treatment of a CM episode rather than as a separate event.

Removal

Removal of a cow (sold or died) after a CM episode can be thought of as the ultimate failure in udder health management. The challenge with this indicator is uncertainty that removal was primarily due to the CM episode, even when the removal record indicates mastitis was the reason. The decision to sell a cow is complex, with a multitude of factors and variation in weighting of those factors across dairies. Nonetheless, evaluation of the proportion of CM episodes removed within a specified number of days after the episode can be informative. It is generally reasonable to assume the sooner a cow is removed after a CM episode the more likely it was the primary reason for removal. Therefore, it is recommended that removal by 7 and 14 days after the CM episode be monitored.

The KPIs to assess outcomes of CM episodes described should all be evaluated as a cohort for a specified period of time. For example, the percentage of CM episodes in a month that resulted in a recurrence should be calculated. Tools to efficiently calculate these indicators are not widely available. Such calculations require handling CM episodes much the way reproductive events are in currently available DMS where a breeding event is updated by a subsequent breeding or pregnancy evaluation event, allowing summary and analysis of the outcomes of breedings. A program allowing efficient summary and analysis of health records (HEALTHSUM) was developed at Washington State University with funding from the US Department of Agriculture.

SUMMARY

Despite a long-standing recognition of the value of records, CM recording standards and the tools for efficient summary and analysis of records are lacking in the industry. Until DMS controls data entry, standard CM recording protocols are needed to ensure accuracy and consistency. These protocols should be based on the 3 simple rules of good recording, and the common issues that compromise record quality detailed in this article should be considered in their development. Accurate and consistent CM records and the ability to efficiently analyze them will be critical to future improvement in udder health management on dairies that have successfully controlled contagious pathogens but struggle with environmental mastitis pathogens.

ACKNOWLEDGMENTS

Funding for work cited was provided by Agriculture and Food Research Initiative Competitive Grant number 2010-85122-20611 from the USDA National Institute of Food and Agriculture.

REFERENCES

1. Hardaker J, Anderson J. Why farm recording systems are doomed to failure. Rev Marketing Agr Econ 1981;49:199–202.
2. Etherington W, Kinsel M, Marsh W. Options in dairy data management. Can Vet J 1995;36:28–33.
3. Kelton D, Bonnett B, Lissemore K. Dairy cattle disease data from secondary databases; use with caution! Proceedings of the European Community Workshop on Genetic Improvement of Functional Traits in Cattle - Health Traits. Interbull Centre, Uppsala, Sweden; 1997. p. 3–10.
4. Giebel S, Wenz J, Poisson S, et al. Implementation of health data entry protocols effect on time for data management. J Dairy Sci 2012;95(Suppl 2):9.
5. Chapinal N, Barrientos A, von Keyserlingk M, et al. Herd-level risk factors for lameness in freestall farms in the northeastern United States and California. J Dairy Sci 2013;96:318–28.
6. Atkinson D, von Keyserlingk M, Weary D. Benchmarking passive transfer of immunity and growth in dairy calves. J Dairy Sci 2017;100:3773–82.
7. Sumner C, von Keyserlingk M, Weary D. How benchmarking motivates farmers to improve dairy calf management. J Dairy Sci 2018;101:3323–33.
8. Thurmond MC. Epidemiologic Methods in Mastitis Treatment and Control. Vet Clin North Am Food Anim Pract 1993;9:435–44.
9. Ruegg PL. Managing mastitis and producing high quality milk. In: Risco C, Melendez P, editors. Dairy production medicine. Hoboken (NJ): John Wiley & Sons, Inc; 2011. p. 207–32.
10. Kelton D, Lissemore K, Martin R. Recommendations for recording and calculating the incidence of selected clinical diseases of dairy cattle. J Dairy Sci 1998;81:2502–9.
11. Schukken Y, Wilson D, Welcome F, et al. Monitoring udder health and milk quality using somatic cell counts. Vet Res 2003;34:579–96.
12. Rhoda D, Pantoja C. Using mastitis records and somatic cell count data. Vet Clin North Am Food Anim Pract 2012;23:347–61.
13. Wenz J. Make the cows the consultants with "good" clinical mastitis recording and analysis. In: Proceedings of the 57st annual conference national mastitis council. Tucson (AZ): NMC; 2018. p. 61–73.
14. Wenz J, Giebel S. Retrospective evaluation of health event data recording on 50 dairies using Dairy Comp 305. J Dairy Sci 2012;95:4699–706.
15. Barkema H, Schukken Y, Lam T, et al. Incidence of clinical mastitis in dairy herds grouped in three categories by bulk milk somatic cell counts. J Dairy Sci 1998;81:411–9.
16. Wenz J, Garry F, Lombard J, et al. Short communication: Efficacy of parenteral ceftiofur for treatment of systemically mild clinical mastitis in dairy cattle. J Dairy Sci 2005;88:3496–9.
17. Schukken Y, Bar D, Hertl J, et al. Correlated time to event data: Modeling repeated clinical mastitis data from dairy cattle in New York State. Prev Vet Med 2010;97:150–6.
18. Hertl J, Schukken Y, Bar D, et al. The effect of recurrent episodes of clinical mastitis caused by gram-positive and gram-negative bacteria and other organisms on mortality and culling in Holstein dairy cows. J Dairy Sci 2011;94:4863–77.
19. Oliveira L, Ruegg P. Treatments of clinical mastitis occurring in cows on 51 large dairy herds in Wisconsin. J Dairy Sci 2014;97:5426–36.

20. Pantoja J, Almeida A, dos Santos B, et al. An investigation of risk factors for two successive cases of clinical mastitis in the same lactation. Livest Sci 2016;194: 10–6.
21. Smith K, Todhunter D, Schoenberger P. Environmental mastitis: cause, prevalence, prevention. J Dairy Sci 1985;68:1531–53.
22. Pinzón-Sánchez C, Ruegg P. Risk factors associated with short-term post-treatment outcomes of clinical mastitis. J Dairy Sci 2011;94:3397–410.
23. Abureema S, Smooker P, Malmo J, et al. Molecular epidemiology of recurrent clinical mastitis due to Streptococcus uberis. J Dairy Sci 2014;97:285–90.

Mammary Gland Immunobiology and Resistance to Mastitis

Lorraine M. Sordillo, MS, PhD

KEYWORDS

• Mastitis • Inflammation • Immunity • Vaccines • Oxylipids • Cytokines

KEY POINTS

- Resistance to the mastitis depends on the efficiency of the mammary gland immune system.
- Mammary gland immunity uses a multifaceted network of physical, cellular, and soluble factors that can be conveniently classified as innate or adaptive immune responses.
- The primary roles of the immune system are to prevent bacterial invasion of the mammary gland, eliminate existing infections, and restore mammary tissues to normal function.
- Strategies to optimize mammary gland defenses can be an effective way to prevent the establishment of new intramammary infections and limit the use of antimicrobials needed to treat mastitis.

INTRODUCTION

The ability of cows to resist the establishment of new intramammary infections depends on the efficiency the mammary gland immune system. The purpose of the immune system is to not only prevent bacterial invasion of the mammary gland but also eliminate existing infections and restore normal tissue function. Components of mammary gland immunity consist of a complex system of tissues, cells, and molecules that work together to defend against a variety of mastitis-causing pathogens. Individual components of the mammary immune system can be generally classified into different functional categories that include the innate and adaptive (or acquired) immune responses. Innate immunity includes a set of resistance mechanisms that can be triggered within seconds to minutes of bacterial challenge. In contrast, the adaptive immune system can take several days to become fully activated and is capable of a

The authors acknowledge research support through grants (2014-68004-21972 and 2017-67015-26676) from the Agriculture and Food Research Initiative Competitive Grants Programs of the USDA National Institute for Food and Agriculture and by an endowment from the Matilda R. Wilson Fund (Detroit, MI).
College of Veterinary Medicine, Michigan State University, 784 Wilson Road, G300 Veterinary Medical Center, East Lansing, MI 48824, USA
E-mail address: sordillo@msu.edu

Vet Clin Food Anim 34 (2018) 507–523
https://doi.org/10.1016/j.cvfa.2018.07.005
0749-0720/18/© 2018 Elsevier Inc. All rights reserved.

vetfood.theclinics.com

more specific response to select bacterial factors that cause mastitis. Although it is convenient to discuss the highly complex nature of mammary gland immunology in terms of innate and adaptive responses, it should be emphasized that these subsystems do not operate independently of each other. It is necessary for both innate and adaptive protective factors of the mammary gland to be highly interactive and coordinated to provide optimal protection from mastitis-causing pathogens.[1] As such, this integrated immune system not only must maintain a delicate balance between activation of defense mechanisms needed to control bacterial pathogenesis during the early stages of infection but also have the capacity to resolve immune activation once the threat of bacterial invasion has passed. This article provides a brief overview of mammary gland immunity, provides examples when the immune system can be compromised, and outlines current strategies to optimize immune responses during times of increased susceptibility to mastitis.

INNATE IMMUNITY

Innate immunity is the initial line of defense when the mammary gland is first exposed to mastitis-causing pathogens. The innate immune response is characterized by a rapid activation that can occur within seconds after initial bacterial exposure. Depending on the efficiency of innate defense mechanisms, mastitis-causing pathogens may be neutralized before any abnormal changes to the milk or mammary tissue occur. Although innate immunity is an immediate line of defense, the recognition and response to bacteria are not highly specific and the immune response is not long lasting. Moreover, innate immune mechanisms are not augmented by repeated exposure to the same mastitis-causing pathogen. The resistance mechanisms of innate immunity can be either localized within affected mammary tissues or quickly recruited from the blood stream to the site of infection after activation by numerous stimuli. Major constituents of innate immunity include the physical barrier of the teat end in addition to a variety of cellular and molecular mechanisms that facilitate protection of the mammary gland (**Table 1**).

Anatomic Defenses

Pathogens must gain entrance to the mammary gland to cause infections, so the teat end is considered the first line of localized defense against mastitis-causing pathogens. The teat end can impede bacterial penetration by several different mechanisms. The teat end has sphincter muscles that surround the teat canal to maintain a tight closure between milkings and hinder bacterial penetration. The teat canal also is lined with a waxy material called keratin that is derived from the epithelial lining. Studies found that accumulation of keratin can provide a physical obstruction to bacteria, particularly during the nonlactating period when the teat canal becomes completely blocked with this substance. Lipid components of keratin also contains antibacterial fatty acid components that have both bacteriostatic and bactericidal activities. In general, gram-positive bacteria are more susceptible than gram-negative bacteria to the bacteriostatic and bactericidal effects of the fatty acids in keratin. Although the proposed mechanisms for keratin's antibacterial activity are still the subject of speculation, there is evidence to suggest that the long chain fatty acids disrupt bacterial lipid membranes, resulting in bacterial cell perforation. Thus, differences in the composition of gram-positive and gram-negative bacterial cell walls may explain the differential antibacterial effects of keratin with respect to bacterial species. More recent evidence suggests that keratin also contains calcium-binding proteins that also may have some antimicrobial activity.[2] Additional studies are justified to better understand the important host-defense capabilities of the teat canal beyond its barrier functions.

Table 1
Predominant innate defense mechanisms of the mammary gland

Factor	Main Functions
Teat end	• Sphincter muscles contract to block bacterial penetration. • Keratin has bacteriostatic activity and forms a barrier. • Furstenberg rosette densely populated with leukocytes, but overall significance is unknown.
Pattern recognition receptors	• Bacterial recognition and activation of inflammatory responses
Complement	• Bacteriolytic and facilitates phagocytosis
Lactoferrin	• Sequestration of iron needed for bacterial growth
Cytokines	• Immunoregulatory for innate immune responses
Oxylipids	• Regulation of microvasculature • Orchestrates proinflammatory and proresolving responses
Epithelial cells	• Pathogen recognition through pattern recognition receptors
Endothelial cells	• Controls of blood flow to affected tissues • Regulates leukocyte migration and activation
Neutrophils	• Phagocytosis and intracellular killing of bacteria through production ROS, antibacterial enzymes, and defensins • NET formation
Macrophages	• Phagocytosis and intracellular killing of bacteria • Production of immunoregulatory cytokines and oxylipids • Removal of cellular debris
Dendritic cells	• Phagocytosis of bacteria • Cytokine production
NK cells	• Target and help eliminate infected host cells • Secretion of antibacterial proteins on activation

Through several complementary mechanisms, the teat end can prevent the penetration of mastitis-causing pathogens and inhibit most bacterial growth. There are some circumstances, however, when this important line of defense is compromised. For example, during the early dry period and just prior to calving, the smooth muscles in the teat canal become more relaxed due to the accumulation of intramammary pressure associated with milk retention. There is also incomplete formation of the keratin lining for up to 2 weeks after the abrupt cessation of lactation that is related directly to increased incidence of mastitis.[3] The teat canal also remains dilated for approximately an hour after milking before muscles can fully contract and may provide another opportunity for bacterial penetration of the teat end. As such, teat antisepsis is an important and widely adopted management practice needed to optimize this initial line of mammary gland defense.

Pathogen Recognition

When mastitis-causing pathogens successfully penetrate the teat end, the ability to sense the presence of bacteria within the mammary gland is an essential for the onset of the innate immune response. Localized mammary cell populations are capable of facilitating pathogen recognition and can effectively stimulate the several immune processes. Both immune and nonimmune cells in the mammary gland possess pattern recognition receptors (PRRs) that can interact with a diverse array of conserved motifs unique to groups of microbes, termed *pathogen-associated molecular patterns (PAMPs).* Examples of these PRRs are the Toll-like receptors (TLRs), which are a family of transmembrane proteins expressed on not only leukocyte populations but also endothelial cells, epithelial cells, and fibroblasts that are distributed throughout mammary tissues.[4,5] Within the TLR family, both TLR-2 and TLR-4 are of particular importance to mammary defense because these receptors recognize PAMPs associated with gram-positive (peptidoglycans) and gram-negative (lipopolysaccharide) mastitis-causing pathogens, including *Staphylococcus aureus*, *Streptococcus uberis*, and *Escherichia coli*.[6,7] After pathogen recognition and binding through PRR-PAMP interactions, intracellular signaling pathways are activated, including nuclear factor (NF)-κB, which control the expression of several soluble mediators that trigger the onset of the inflammatory cascade.[8]

Onset of Inflammation

Inflammation is a critical component of the innate defense system that should eliminate bacteria within the mammary gland, assist with the repair of any tissue damage that may occur during bacterial invasion, and restore normal tissue structure and function. The inflammatory cascade results not only in the accumulation of antimicrobial factors in the milk but also the increased movement of peripheral blood leukocytes and other plasma components from the blood and into the mammary gland.[1] An efficient mammary gland inflammatory response generally should last less than a week and not cause any noticeable change to milk or mammary tissues. Dysfunctional mammary inflammatory cascades that become exaggerated or protracted, however, can result in extensive tissue damage resulting in uncontrolled acute or chronic mastitis that contribute to significant milk production losses.[1,9,10] Thus, mammary gland inflammatory responses should have a rapid onset to neutralize bacteria during the initial stages of tissue invasio, but a timely resolution to avoid the immunopathology associated with mastitis (**Fig. 1**).

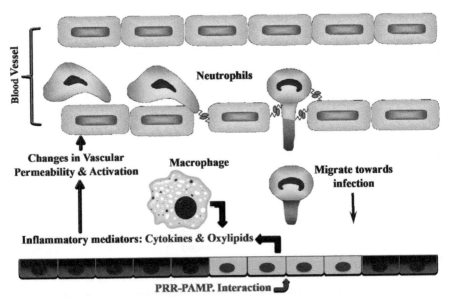

Fig. 1. Major stages associated with the onset of inflammation.

The activation of NF-κB is a major signaling pathway by which soluble mediators are produced to drive the onset of the mammary inflammatory cascade.[11,12] Cytokines are one of the principal soluble mediators produced during all stages of the inflammatory response. Cytokines are a heterogeneous group of low-molecular-weight glycoproteins secreted by both immune and nonimmune cells with the capacity to regulate many different aspects of the immune response, including inflammation. There are several different cytokine categories based on their structure, function, and origin that include interleukins (ILs), interferons (IFNs), chemokines, colony-stimulating factors (CSFs), and tumor necrosis factors (TNFs).

Cytokines bind to receptors on target cell membranes and can exert an autocrine, paracrine, or endocrine action. Individual cytokines can interact with other cytokines synergistically, additively, or antagonistically on multiple cellular targets. For example, TNF-α and IL-1β are expressed rapidly during the initial stages of infection and have potent proinflammatory functions whereas IL4, IL-10, and IL-17 actively promote the resolution of the inflammatory cascade.[11] Most cytokines have very short half-lives, so their synthesis and function usually occur in bursts of activity. Cytokines regulate the intensity and duration of the host response to infection by regulating (enhancing or inhibiting) the activation, proliferation, and differentiation of cells involved in the immune response. With respect to the inflammatory response, cytokines are essential to facilitate the extravasation of leukocytes from the blood stream and to the site of bacterial invasion in mammary tissues.

Another important group of inflammatory signaling molecules is a family of potent lipid-derived mediators referred to as oxylipids, also known as oxylipins or eicosanoids in the literature. These potent lipid mediators are derived from polyunsaturated fatty acids and are capable of regulating essentially every aspect of the initiation and resolution of the inflammatory response.[13,14] Whereas many immune and nonimmune cell populations are capable of producing oxylipids, macrophages and endothelial cells are a major cellular source within most tissues, including the mammary gland.[15,16] Oxylipid biosynthesis is initiated when macrophages or endothelial cells come into contact with PAMPs or other inflammatory stimuli, such as cytokines. Within minutes of exposure to these proinflammatory agonists, polyunsaturated fatty acids are liberated from phospholipids located in cellular or nuclear membranes through the actions of phospholipases. These fatty acid substrates are then oxidized nonenzymatically by reactive oxygen species (ROS) or through different enzymatic routes, including cyclooxygenase (COX), lipoxygenase (LOX), and cytochrome P450 pathways to produce a variety oxylipids that can either enhance or resolve the inflammatory cascade.[16] A majority of early studies investigating the role of oxylipids in mammary gland inflammatory responses focused solely on the arachidonic acid–derived eicosanoids derived from the COX pathway, such as the prostaglandins (PGs), thromboxanes (TX), and leukotrienes (LT).[17,18] The recent advent of highly sensitive lipidomic technologies, however, has enabled the identification of a complex network of oxylipids that may be produced from different polyunsaturated fatty acid substrates and oxygenated by different pathways.[16] To date, there are more than 130 oxylipids that have been identified and many characterized for their biological activities.[19]

Depending on the type of invading mastitis-causing pathogen, the amount and timing of initial soluble mediator production can vary considerably. For example, the expressions of cytokine transcripts were greater and expressed more rapidly in *Escherichia coli*–infected mammary glands compared with *Staphylococcus aureus* mastitis.[20] The severity of mastitis also may be associated with specific inflammatory mediator profiles, such as excessively high concentrations of TNF-α during severe acute coliform mastitis.[21] Moreover, previous studies showed that TXB2 and PGE2, known proinflammatory oxylipids, may have important roles in the enhanced severity of *E coli* mastitis that occurs during the periparturient period.[22] Previous studies also showed that increased biosynthesis of PGE2 was related to bacterial growth and systemic disease severity during *E coli* mastitis.[23] Inflammation is primarily a reaction of the microcirculation where both cytokines and oxylipids have the capacity to interact directly with blood vessels in the mammary gland to alter vascular tone and blood flow within the affected tissues, increase vasodilation of capillaries, and increase vascular permeability needed for the migration of blood leukocytes to the site of injury.[15] The collective responses of the vascular endothelium and infiltration of blood leukocytes into affected tissues as a consequence of cytokine and oxylipid biosynthesis can result in some of the classic signs of inflammation that include heat, swelling, redness, pain, and loss of function.

Innate Cellular Defenses

During inflammation, both resident and newly recruited mammary gland leukocytes play an essential role during the early stages of pathogenesis. Within uninfected mammary tissues, lymphocytes and macrophages are the predominant leukocyte types with relatively low numbers of neutrophils. Total somatic cell counts (SCCs) in healthy mammary glands are often less than 10^5 cells/mL of milk, and the distribution of leukocytes varies as a function of lactation stage. Total SCCs can increase to greater than 10^6 cells/mL of milk within just a few hours of bacterial invasion, however, and the major leukocyte type during inflammation are neutrophils. The influx of neutrophil is initiated by cytokines and oxylipids that act directly on the vasculature to cause reductions in blood velocity with a concomitant increase in the expression of adhesion molecules on endothelial cells.[15] Adhesion molecules on leukocytes attach to vascular adhesion molecules to facilitate the migration of leukocytes from the blood to the site of injury.[24,25] Neutrophils first marginate and then adhere to the local endothelium near the site of infection. Cytokines, oxylipids, and other mediator molecules stimulate adherent neutrophils to move between endothelial cells and pass the basement membrane into the damaged tissue areas.[1,15] The movement of neutrophils within the tissues is facilitated by chemotactic gradients created by inflammatory mediator molecules at the localized site of infection. Neutrophil migration can occur quickly and accumulate within affected tissues as soon as 30 minutes to 60 minutes after injury.[26] The promptness and magnitude of neutrophil migration into mammary gland tissues and milk are considered major determining factors for the establishment of new intramammary infections.[27]

An important innate defense mechanism facilitated by mammary gland leukocytes is the ingestion and killing of bacteria, a process referred to as phagocytosis. In the mammary gland, phagocytosis is carried out primarily by neutrophils and macrophages, but dendritic cells are also capable of phagocytosis. The phagocytic process involves the engulfment of bacteria, where it is then encapsulated within a cytoplasmic vacuole called a phagolysosome. Neutrophils can kill phagocytosed bacterial by either oxygen-dependent or protein-mediated mechanisms. The oxygen-dependent system is operative during the ingestion process in which there is a major burst of oxidative metabolism. The increased oxygen consumption results in the production of reactive oxygen and nitrogen intermediates that are produced through a metabolic process known as respiratory burst. These microbicidal oxidizing agents are located within phagolysosomes and can oxidize bacterial membrane lipids and cause the pathogen's destruction. The primary enzymes involved in catalyzing the oxidation process are myeloperoxidase and superoxide dismutase.[1,27]

In addition, bacteria may become exposed to and destroyed by several oxygen-independent reactants, including lysozyme, a variety of cationic proteins, and lactoferrin. These antimicrobial elements of neutrophils also are stored within large cytoplasmic granules unique to bovine neutrophils. For example, several cationic peptides have been isolated from these large granules of bovine neutrophils and have been studied and described experimentally. Bovine neutrophil cationic proteins are a heterogeneous group including cathelicidin family members and the β-defensins that display antibacterial activity against pathogens associated with mammary gland infection. The degraded bacteria are then exocytosed from the neutrophil with minimal collateral damage to mammary tissues. Mammary gland neutrophils can ingest fat, casein, and other milk components that render them less effective at phagocytosizing bacteria. The phagocytic and bactericidal activities of these cells are especially diminished during the periparturient period and are believed an underlying cause of increased susceptibility to mastitis during this stage of lactation. The phagocytic and bactericidal capabilities of neutrophils, however, can be increased substantially in the presence of opsonic antibody for specific pathogens.[27,28]

Neutrophil extracellular trap (NET) formation is an additional antimicrobial defense mechanism in the innate immune system. Pathogen stimulation of neutrophils triggers the release of nuclear material (DNA and histones) as well as granular proteins and extracellular fibers that function to trap and kill microbes. Studies suggest that NETs provide highly concentrated foci of antibacterial substances that bind and kill bacteria independently of phagocytic uptake in the mammary gland.[29,30] NETs also may serve as a physical barrier that prevents further spread of bacteria throughout a cow's tissues. NET formation may be of particular importance to the mammary gland due to their ability to function in the presence of milk in contrast to other neutrophil functions that can be suppressed in that environment.[30]

Natural killer (NK) cells are a subpopulation of lymphocytes that also may play an important role as part of mammary gland innate immunity. They are characterized as large granular lymphocytes that have cytotoxic activity independent of the major histocompatibility complex (MHC). A unique aspect of NK cells is their ability to use Fc receptors to participate in antibody-dependent, cell-mediated cytotoxicity. Cytokine-stimulated NK cells also are capable of killing bacteria by releasing bactericidal proteins. NK cells isolated from bovine mammary tissue exhibit bactericidal activity against *S aureus* and, therefore, these lymphoid populations could be an important aspect of innate defense in preventing mastitis. Changes in this cell population during the periparturient period have not been studied extensively, but the potent bactericidal activity of these cells makes them worthy of future study.[3]

Innate Soluble Defenses

In addition to the antibacterial functions of mammary leukocyte populations, bacteria may be exposed to and destroyed by protein-mediated defense mechanisms. Lactoferrin, for example, is among the best-characterized antimicrobial proteins and is the most common iron-binding protein found in the exocrine secretions of mammals. Lactoferrin concentrations in milk fluctuate during the lactation cycle with the highest concentrations observed in the fully involuted gland. The ability of lactoferrin, in the presence of bicarbonate, to bind soluble iron in milk is the basis of its most important biological activities. Lactoferrin can act as a transport protein by moving the bound iron to a different area within the host. In addition, the iron-binding capability of lactoferrin greatly reduces soluble ferric iron available to multiplying bacteria. Withholding this essential element prevents the production of dismutase, an enzyme produced by bacteria to counteract superoxide radicals generated by the host. Collectively, the iron-binding capacity of lactoferrin results in a bacteriostatic effect, resulting in greatly reduced bacterial multiplication rates. Lactoferrin also can have direct bactericidal effects on certain mastitis-causing pathogens and is known to play a role in normal lymphocyte and macrophage functions. The bacteriostatic and antibacterial properties of lactoferrin, however, are depressed in the presence of citrate, a natural buffer produced by the mammary epithelium, which chelates iron into a form that bacteria can utilize. Citrate levels in milk tend to be very low during involution but increase substantially at calving. There exists a direct correlation between changes in citrate and lactoferrin ratios in lacteal secretions and susceptibility to new intramammary infections.[1,3]

There are several other soluble factors associated with innate mammary gland defenses. Complement is a collection of proteins present in serum and milk, which can have an impact on both innate and adaptive immunity. Many of the biological activities of complement are mediated through complement receptors located on a variety of cells. Complement activation can occur through 3 different pathways resulting in lysis of bacterial target cells. Gram-negative bacteria, such as *E coli*, are especially sensitive to complement-mediated lysis. Complement also functions in concert with a specific antibody as an opsonin, which promotes bacterial phagocytosis and intracellular killing by neutrophils and macrophages. Concentrations of complement are highest in colostrum, inflamed mammary glands, and during involution. In contrast, concentrations of complement are lowest during lactation. Therefore, because of its intermittent presence in milk, complement is believed to play only a minor bactericidal role in the mammary gland.[28]

Resolution of Inflammation

As outlined previously, the onset of inflammation to bacterial invasion is a complex and tightly regulated response. Whereas a rapid and robust inflammatory response is protective, an uncontrolled acute or chronic inflammatory reaction can lead to extensive tissue damage that is associated with diseases pathogenesis. Therefore, a timely and natural resolution of inflammation is fundamental to overall health of the mammary gland. The resolution of inflammation is an active event involving specific proresolving pathways and mediators that expedite the shutdown process by limiting leukocyte infiltration into affected tissues, modifying soluble mediator production, removal of cellular debris, and repairing damaged tissues.[31,32] An essential requirement to turn off the inflammatory response is the removal of the mastitis-causing pathogens that initiated the inflammatory cascade. The successful neutralization of the inciting pathogen signals the cessation of proinflammatory mediator synthesis and leads to their catabolism. Alternatively, the production of several anti-inflammatory or proresolving soluble mediators is enhanced. Therefore, if neutrophils are able to migrate rapidly from the blood stream to the mammary gland and effectively eliminate the bacteria, then the recruitment of leukocytes should cease and milk SCCs return to levels found in healthy cows. If bacteria persist, however, then the inflammatory response continues into an acute or chronic state. Prolonged and/or excessive migration of leukocytes from the blood causes considerable damage to mammary parenchymal tissues that result in reduced milk production.

Both cytokines and oxylipids are critical soluble mediators that play a central role in the resolution of the inflammatory cascade. As discussed previously, IL-4, IL-10, and IL-17 are known to actively promote the resolution of inflammation in the mammary gland.[11] The expression of these anti-inflammatory cytokines depends on the leukocyte profiles within mammary tissues and the degree of activation based on the infection status of the mammary gland. The precise role of cytokines in orchestrated mammary gland inflammatory processes have been well documented over the past several decades.[1,15] A new area of research into the termination of inflammation, however, is the production of lipid mediators with potent anti-inflammatory and proresolving activities. Studies conducted in human and laboratory species showed that the resolution of inflammation is an active process governed by several distinct families of proresolving oxylipids, which include resolvins, protectins, and lipoxins (LXs).[33] Although some metabolites derived from the cyclooxygenase (COX) pathway traditionally were associated with triggering the onset of the inflammatory response, there are several COX-derived metabolites, including PGD_2, PGJ_2, and 15-deoxy-PGJ_2, which have the capacity to suppress various proinflammatory signaling pathways. There is also considerable evidence to suggest that certain PGs produced during the onset of inflammation, such as PGE_2, can serve as negative feedback signals to facilitate the resolution of inflammation.[34] The active biosynthesis of proresolving lipid mediators plays an essential role in limiting neutrophil infiltration into affected tissues, enhancing macrophage clearance of apoptotic cells within affected tissues, and facilitates the restoration of tissues to normal function.[32] Unfortunately, there is not a great deal of in vivo research available in dairy cattle to suggest how proresolving or anti-inflammatory oxylipids may contribute to the resolution of mammary gland inflammatory responses.[16] The relative expression of plasma oxylipids with known roles in the resolution of inflammation was reported to decrease in transition cows when biomarkers of inflammation are often enhanced.[35] Previous studies reported an imbalance between anti-inflammatory (LXA4) and proinflammatory (LTB4) oxylipids in cows with chronic mastitis due to lower concentrations of LXA4 in the milk.[36] A broader understanding of how oxylipids profiles shift to facilitate both the onset and resolution of inflammation is required to design efficacious intervention strategies to optimize bovine inflammatory responses especially during times of increased susceptibility to disease.

ADAPTIVE IMMUNITY

Although adaptive immunity takes longer than innate immunity to develop after microbial exposure, it becomes increasingly important if pathogens are able to evade or are not completely eliminated by the innate defense system. In contrast to the generalized nature of innate immunity, adaptive immunity is able to elicit immune responses to specific factors associated with bacterial pathogens, which are referred to as antigens. A fascinating feature of the adaptive immune system is the ability of a cow to recognize and respond to billions of unique antigens they may encounter. When an antigen is encountered more than one time, a heightened state of immune reactivity occurs as a consequence of immunologic memory. As such, a memory response is much faster, considerably stronger, lasts longer, and often is more effective in clearing pathogens compared with the initial exposure to a particular antigen. The ability of the adaptive immune responses to be amplified by repeated exposure to a particular pathogen provides the foundation of mastitis vaccine strategies. It also is important that inappropriate specific immune responses do not occur against a cow's own antigens. For this reason, the immune system is able to distinguish self from nonself and selectively react to only foreign antigens. The ability to recognize only foreign antigens is mediated by genetically diverse, membrane-bound proteins, called MHC molecules. A specific immune response only occurs if antigens are combined with an MHC molecule on the surface of certain cells, a process referred to as antigen presentation. Major components of the innate immune system include immunoglobulin (Ig) molecules, macrophages, dendritic cells, and several different lymphoid populations that mediate recognition of specific pathogenic factors.

Adaptive Cellular Defenses

Generation of effective specific immunity involves 2 broad cell types, including lymphocytes and antigen-presenting cells. Lymphocytes recognize bacterial antigens through membrane receptors specific to the invading pathogen. These are the cells that mediate the defining attributes of adaptive immunity, including specificity, diversity, memory, and self/nonself recognition. The T cells and B cells are distinct subsets of lymphocytes that differ in function and the expression profiles of protein products. The T cells can be further subdivided into $\alpha\beta$ T cells, which include CD4$^+$ (helper T [T_H]) and CD8$^+$ (T-cytotoxic [Tc]) cells and $\gamma\delta$ T cells. The T_H cells can be refined further based on functional groupings that include T_H1, T_H2, T_H17, and regulatory T cells (Tregs) (**Table 2**). Depending on the stage of lactation and tissue location, the percentages of these cells can vary significantly.[1]

The T_H cells produce cytokines in response to recognition of antigen-MHC complexes on antigen-presenting cells (B cells, macrophages, and dendritic cells). When activated, the variety of immunoregulatory cytokines produced by T_H cells play an important role in activating both T cell and B cells, macrophages, neutrophils, and various other cells that participate in the immune response. Differences in the particular pattern of cytokines produced by activated T_H cells results in different types of immune responses. For example, IFN-γ and IL-2 are believed to enhance some cellular activities associated with innate immunity, such as phagocytosis and intracellular killing. Alternatively, these same cytokines may also enhance the proliferation and differentiation of T cells and B cells during adaptive immune responses.[1,3]

Table 2
Predominant adaptive defense mechanisms of the mammary gland

Factor	Main Functions
MHC	• Distinguishes host molecules from foreign molecules
Dendritic cells	• Antigen presentation • Cytokine production
Macrophages	• Antigen presentation • Cytokine production
$\alpha\beta$ T cells	• T_H cells (T_H1, T_H 2, T_H17, Treg); produce cytokines that regulate adaptive immunity • Role in Ig isotype switching • Tc cells; lysis of damaged host cells • Produce cytokines capable of down-regulating leukocyte functions
$\gamma\delta$ T cells	• Prevalent in ruminants and found at mucosal surfaces • Role in the mammary gland is speculative
B cells	• Mature B cells are antigen-presenting cells and expand into antigen-specific memory cells • Plasma cells synthesize and secrete antigen-specific antibodies
Ig (antibodies)	• IgM is the largest and first produced; role in agglutination and complement activation • IgG1 is selectively transported into the mammary secretion; enhances bacterial phagocytosis through opsonization • IgG2 is transported into the mammary gland during neutrophil influx; opsonizes bacteria and enhances phagocytosis • IgA is found at mucosal surfaces and has antiviral function
Cytokines	• Immunoregulatory for adaptive immunity • Facilitates leukocyte functional capacity

The cytotoxic functions of Tc cells include the recognize and eliminate altered foreign antigens when presented in conjunction with MHC class I molecules. In the mammary gland, Tc cells are believed to protect mammary epithelial cells against intracellular pathogens once the microbial antigens are exposed on the cell surface. There is some speculation that Tc cells also may act as scavengers that remove old or damaged secretory cells in the mammary gland. Similar to the T_H cells, suppressor functions of Tc cells are believed to control or modulate the immune response by the repertoire of cytokines that they produce. The suppressor functions of Tc cells can become activated in infected mammary glands or during the periparturient period and may contribute to impaired local defenses under these circumstances.[3]

The biological functions of $\gamma\delta$ T cells have been the subject of much speculation. Their functions are primarily associated with the protection of epithelial surfaces. There are indications that $\gamma\delta$ T cells can mediate cytotoxicity with variable involvement of MHC class I molecules.[37] These cells also may play a role in infectious diseases and, therefore, provide an important line of defense against bacterial diseases, such as mastitis. Mammary secretions and tissue express a higher percentage of $\gamma\delta$ T cells compared with the peripheral blood. The fact that the percentages of these cells decrease significantly in the mammary gland during times of increased susceptibility to disease suggests that these lymphocytes may constitute an essential line of defense against mastitis-causing pathogens.

The primary role of B cells is to produce antibodies, also called Igs, against invading pathogens. B cells use membrane bound antibody molecules to recognize specific pathogens. After recognition, B cells can internalize, process, and present antigen in the context of MHC class II molecules to T_H cells. The T_H cells become activated and begin to secrete certain cytokines, including IL-2, which in turn induce proliferation and differentiation of the B cells into antibody producing plasma cells or memory B cells. In contrast to T_H cells, the percentages of B cells remain fairly constant between stages of lactation.

Macrophages are a predominant cell type found in the milk and tissues of healthy, involuted, and lactating mammary glands. Whereas these cells have a role in early innate immune responses, such as phagocytes and production of inflammatory mediators, macrophages also play a key role in antigen processing and presentation. Antigens from ingested bacteria are processed within macrophages and appear on the cell surface in association with MHC class II molecules. When a naive T_H cell encounters antigen complexed with MHC class II molecules, it can proliferate and differentiate into memory cells and cytokine-producing effector cells, as described previously.

Adaptive Humoral Defenses

Antibodies function as the soluble effector of the humoral component of the adaptive immune response. Antigen-activated B cells proliferate and differentiate into antibody-secreting plasma cells. Antibodies in lacteal secretions are synthesized locally or are selectively transported from serum. Four classes of antibodies, or Igs, are known to influence mammary gland defense against mastitis-causing bacteria and include IgG_1, IgG_2, IgA, and IgM. Each of these classes differs in physiochemical and biological properties. The concentration of each Ig class in mammary secretion varies depending on stage of lactation and infection status of the mammary gland. In healthy glands, the concentration of Ig is low during lactation but slowly increases during the nonlactating periods and reaches peak concentrations during colostrogenesis. High concentrations of Ig also occur in the mammary gland during inflammation. The concentration of Ig in the gland is dependent on the degree of permeability of secretory tissue and the number of Ig-producing cells that are present in the mammary gland.[1]

STRATEGIES TO OPTIMIZE MAMMARY GLAND IMMUNITY

Although the mammary gland is equipped with a diverse and highly interactive network of innate and adaptive immune mechanisms, there are certain times in a cow's production cycle when the mammary immune system is compromised resulting in higher rates of new intramammary infections. Research over the past several decades suggests that many aspects of the innate and adaptive immunity are especially compromised in periparturient dairy cows. Dysfunctional immune responsiveness around the time of calving is considered the major underlying factor that explains why periparturient cows are susceptible to so many different metabolic and infectious diseases, including mastitis. The development of innovative strategies that can enhance otherwise impaired mammary gland immune responses during periods of increased disease susceptibility could have a major impact on the incidence of mastitis.

Dietary Supplements

The nutritional status of dairy cattle, especially during the periparturient period, is directly related to the efficiency of the immune response.[38] Nutritional requirements of cows fluctuate throughout the production cycle and any mismanagement of dietary requirements has an adverse impact on immunity and disease resistance. Meeting the nutritional requirements of the periparturient cow is especially challenging because of the increased dietary demands associated with the onset of copious milk synthesis and secretion with a concomitant decline in dry matter intake after calving. As a consequence, early lactation cows experience severe negative energy and protein balance, which is directly related to dysfunction inflammatory reactions. Altered nutrient metabolism, dysfunctional inflammatory responses, and increased incidence and severity of oxidative stress around the time of calving can form destructive feedback loops to compromise the overall immune system in periparturient cows.[39]

Although the interaction between nutrient metabolism and immunity is complex and not completely understood at this time, the need for a balanced supply of dietary micronutrients (vitamins and trace mineral) is widely recognized as having an essential role in optimizing immune responses and increasing disease resistance around the time of calving. The significance of micronutrients in supporting essential immune responses was best illustrated in dairy cattle with overt deficiencies in certain vitamins and minerals during the periparturient period that resulted in increased incidence and severity of mastitis.[40] Most of the current information on micronutrients and their immunoregulatory properties in controlling mastitis focuses on selenium (Se), vitamin E, vitamin A, copper, and zinc. Of all of these micronutrients, vitamin E and Se are the best characterized with respect to their role in supporting aspects of the innate and adaptive immune responses that can influence mastitis susceptibility. For example, supplementation of cows with both vitamin E and Se improved the functional capabilities of bovine neutrophils compared with neutrophils isolated from cows with marginal of overt deficiencies in these micronutrients. Supplementing cows with vitamin E and Se around during late gestation to avoid deficiencies after calving was proved to effectively reduce the incidence and severity of clinical mastitis while also preventing the establishment of new intramammary infections during the early lactating period.[41,42] Based on these early studies, it is now a common practice to supplement dairy cattle during the late dry period before deficiencies are likely to develop as the cow approaches calving. There also exist compelling data to suggest that vitamin A, copper, and zinc have significant immunoregulatory functions that can optimize innate and adaptive immune responses needed for improved mastitis resistance.[38] A common mechanism by which most of these micronutrients function is through their antioxidant properties and protecting immune cell populations from the toxic effects of ROS. The primary function of antioxidants is to delay, prevent, or remove oxidative damage to cellular macromolecules, such as membrane phospholipids. During an inflammatory response, neutrophils and macrophage produce large quantities of ROS with the purpose of killing invading bacteria. For the ROS not to cause bystander damage to the cows own cells, it is important that adequate amounts of antioxidants are provided by the diet so that they can be incorporated into mammary gland tissues and immune cell populations.[38] The key to ensuring dairy cattle consume adequate amounts of these important micronutrients is by directly testing animals at the herd level to detect any patterns of overall nutrient deficiencies. Supplementing the diets of cows with recommended doses of vitamins and minerals is a practical means of enhancing mammary gland immunity and reducing the incidence of mastitis.

Immunomodulators

Strategies to optimize host immunity during times of increased disease susceptibility with biological response modifiers is an area of research that was explored extensively. Cytokines are one class of immunomodulators that were investigated for their capacity to enhance bovine immune responses and to reduce or prevent intramammary infections.[3] Because cytokines play a central role in orchestrating immunity, administering the recombinant form of these immunomodulators during times when normal cytokine expression is compromised seemed a logical approach to enhance disease resistance. The recombinant cytokines studies to date include IL-1, IL-2, granulocyte-CSF (G-CSF), and IFN-γ. The available data provide convincing evidence that these recombinant cytokines can enhance the functional capabilities of cells involved in both innate and adaptive immunity. For example, IFN-γ, G-CSF, and IL-1 were effective in increasing neutrophil migration to the mammary gland and enhancing the bactericidal activity of these important cells of the innate immune response.[3] Both IFN-γ and IL-2 also were able of enhancing T-cell responses to specific antigen with the suggestion that these cytokines may be effective mastitis vaccine adjuvants.[1,11] As with any intervention strategy, however, the key to effective translation of experimental findings to practical on farm application is to clearly define the threshold between therapeutic and toxic doses of these potent immunomodulators. Because cytokines activity is short lived, strategies that could enhance the pharmacodynamic response of the recombinant preparations are essential for practical utility in a dairy farm setting. In addressing this need, the recombinant form of bovine G-CSF was covalently bound to a water-soluble polymer that would extend the duration of cytokine activity needed to achieve therapeutic benefits. A single dose of the PEGylated bovine G-CSF (pegbovigrastim) administered approximately 7 days prior to calving and again on the day of calving was efficacious in reducing the incidence of clinical mastitis during early lactation.[43] There is now a commercially available PEGylated bovine G-CSF (Imrestor, Elanco, Greenfield, IN) that is used in the field to overcome compromised neutrophil migration and activation during the periparturient period. The use of novel cytokine formulations, such as pegbovigrastim, seems a novel approach to overcome periparturient immune dysfunction and reduced susceptibility to clinical mastitis.

Target	Type and Route of Administration	Commercial Name
Coliforms	Bacterin; subcutaneous at dry off, 30 d later, and within 14 d of calving	Enviracor J-5, Zoetis (Parsippany, New Jersey)
Coliforms	Bacterin; subcutaneous at dry off and again 2–4 wk later	J-Vac, Merial (Duluth, GA)
Coliforms	Bacterin-toxoid; intramuscular at dry off and 2–4 wk pos calving	Endovac-Bovi, Immvac (Columbia, MO)
S. aureus	Bacterin; intramuscular with a booster after 14 d	Lysigin, Boehringer Ingelheim Vetmedica (Duluth, Georgia)
S aureus Coliform	Bacterin and polyvalent containing E coli J5 and S aureus; intramuscular with a booster after 14 d	Startvac, Hipra, Spain
Mycoplasma bovis	Bacterin; subcutaneous in 2 doses at 2–4 wk intervals	Myomune, BioImmune (Scottsdale, AZ)

Table 3
Available commercial mastitis vaccines

MASTITIS VACCINES

The primary goals of any vaccination program are to develop specific immune response against a pathogenic agent, prevent the establishment of new infections, and diminish the pathologic consequences of infections that do occur. Vaccines that can effectively prevent new infections have the added benefit of mitigating the spread of contagious pathogens throughout the herd and reducing the need of antimicrobials to treat mastitis. The immunologic basis of mastitis vaccines is to stimulate the adaptive immune response to specific antigenic determinants. In doing so, a vaccine has the potential to enhance cell-mediated immunity directed against certain mastitis pathogens and to increase specific antibodies in both blood and milk. Over the past several decades, some progress has been made to development of commercial, herd-specific autovaccines and other experimental vaccines. Most previous efforts in vaccine development have targeted S aureus or E coli mastitis. Less emphasis has been placed on assessing the possibility of developing vaccine strategies for streptococcal and mycoplasma.[44,45] **Table 3** is a summary of some currently available commercial mastitis vaccines. The efficacy and economic benefits of using mastitis vaccine continues to be a subject of debate due to the variable findings in the scientific literature concerning the ability to prevent new intramammary infections or reduce the severity of disease, especially in herds with high rates of mastitis.[44] The most practical use for vaccines in any mastitis control program likely will be in conjunction with other known control strategies based on excellent milking hygiene, teat dipping, segregation, and culling of chronically infected cows.

SUMMARY

Dairy cattle are especially susceptible to mastitis during certain stages of the lactation cycle. The frequency of new intramammary infections is greatest during the early dry period and lower in the fully involuted mammary gland and dramatically increases during the periparturient period. Changes in the incidence of mastitis with respect to lactation stage are directly related to changes in the composition, magnitude, and efficiency of the mammary gland defense system. The development of innovative strategies that can enhance an otherwise impaired immune response during periods of increased susceptibility to disease could have a major impact on the incidence of mastitis. The challenge that confronts researchers now is to gain a better understanding of the complex interactions between the pathogenesis of bacteria, host responses needed to eliminate the pathogens from the mammary gland, and methods to enhance the immune potential of these factors before disease is established.

REFERENCES

1. Aitken SL, Corl CM, Sordillo LM. Immunopathology of mastitis: insights into disease recognition and resolution. J Mammary Gland Biol Neoplasia 2011;16(4): 291–304.
2. Smolenski GA, Cursons RT, Hine BC, et al. Keratin and S100 calcium-binding proteins are major constituents of the bovine teat canal lining. Vet Res 2015;46:113.
3. Sordillo LM, Streicher KL. Mammary gland immunity and mastitis susceptibility. J Mammary Gland Biol Neoplasia 2002;7(2):135–46.
4. Jungi TW, Farhat K, Burgener IA, et al. Toll-like receptors in domestic animals. Cell Tissue Res 2011;343(1):107–20.
5. Kumar H, Kawai T, Akira S. Pathogen recognition by the innate immune system. Int Rev Immunol 2011;30.
6. Goldammer T, Zerbe H, Molenaar A, et al. Mastitis increases mammary mRNA abundance of beta-defensin 5, toll-like-receptor 2 (TLR2), and TLR4 but not TLR9 in cattle. Clin Diagn Lab Immunol 2004;11(1):174–85.
7. Porcherie A, Cunha P, Trotereau A, et al. Repertoire of Escherichia coli agonists sensed by innate immunity receptors of the bovine udder and mammary epithelial cells. Vet Res 2012;43(1):14.
8. Liang Y, Zhou Y, Shen P. NF-kappaB and its regulation on the immune system. Cell Mol Immunol 2004;1(5):343–50.
9. Akers RM, Nickerson SC. Mastitis and its impact on structure and function in the ruminant mammary gland. J Mammary Gland Biol Neoplasia 2011;16(4):275–89.
10. Halasa T, Huijps K, Osteras O, et al. Economic effects of bovine mastitis and mastitis management: a review. Vet Q 2007;29(1):18–31.
11. Bannerman DD. Pathogen-dependent induction of cytokines and other soluble inflammatory mediators during intramammary infection of dairy cows. J Anim Sci 2009;87(13 Suppl):10–25.
12. Boulanger D, Bureau F, Melotte D, et al. Increased nuclear factor kappaB activity in milk cells of mastitis-affected cows. J Dairy Sci 2003;86(4):1259–67.
13. Mattmiller SA, Carlson BA, Sordillo LM. Regulation of inflammation by selenium and selenoproteins: impact on eicosanoid biosynthesis. J Nutr Sci 2013;2:e28.
14. Serhan CN, Chiang N. Endogenous pro-resolving and anti-inflammatory lipid mediators: a new pharmacologic genus. Br J Pharmacol 2008;153(Suppl 1): S200–15.
15. Ryman VE, Packiriswamy N, Sordillo LM. Role of endothelial cells in bovine mammary gland health and disease. Anim Health Res Rev 2015;16(2):135–49.
16. Sordillo LM. Symposium review: Oxylipids and the regulation of bovine mammary inflammatory responses. J Dairy Sci 2018;101(6):5629–41.
17. Atroshi F, Sankari S, Rizzo A, et al. Prostaglandins, glutathione metabolism, and lipid peroxidation in relation to inflammation in bovine mastitis. Adv Exp Med Biol 1990;264:203–7.
18. Zia S, Giri SN, Cullor J, et al. Role of eicosanoids, histamine, and serotonin in the pathogenesis of Klebsiella pneumoniae-induced bovine mastitis. Am J Vet Res 1987;48(11):1617–25.

19. Wang Y, Armando AM, Quehenberger O, et al. Comprehensive ultra-performance liquid chromatographic separation and mass spectrometric analysis of eicosanoid metabolites in human samples. J Chromatogr A 2014;1359:60–9.

20. Lee JW, Bannerman DD, Paape MJ, et al. Characterization of cytokine expression in milk somatic cells during intramammary infections with Escherichia coli or Staphylococcus aureus by real-time PCR. Vet Res 2006;37(2):219–29.

21. Sordillo LM, Peel JE. Effect of interferon-gamma on the production of tumor necrosis factor during acute Escherichia coli mastitis. J Dairy Sci 1992;75(8):2119–25.

22. Vangroenweghe F, Duchateau L, Boutet P, et al. Effect of carprofen treatment following experimentally induced Escherichia coli mastitis in primiparous cows. J Dairy Sci 2005;88(7):2361–76.

23. Pezeshki A, Stordeur P, Wallemacq H, et al. Variation of inflammatory dynamics and mediators in primiparous cows after intramammary challenge with Escherichia coli. Vet Res 2011;42(1):15.

24. Hodgkinson AJ, Carpenter EA, Smith CS, et al. Adhesion molecule expression in the bovine mammary gland. Vet Immunol Immunopathol 2007;115(3–4):205–15.

25. Maddox JF, Aherne KM, Reddy CC, et al. Increased neutrophil adherence and adhesion molecule mRNA expression in endothelial cells during selenium deficiency. J Leukoc Biol 1999;65(5):658–64.

26. Summers C, Rankin SM, Condliffe AM, et al. Neutrophil kinetics in health and disease. Trends Immunol 2010;31(8):318–24.

27. Paape MJ, Shafer-Weaver K, Capuco AV, et al. Immune surveillance of mammary tissue by phagocytic cells. Adv Exp Med Biol 2000;480:259–77.

28. Rainard P, Riollet C. Innate immunity of the bovine mammary gland. Vet Res 2006;37(3):369–400.

29. Grinberg N, Elazar S, Rosenshine I, et al. Beta-hydroxybutyrate abrogates formation of bovine neutrophil extracellular traps and bactericidal activity against mammary pathogenic Escherichia coli. Infect Immun 2008;76(6):2802–7.

30. Lippolis JD, Reinhardt TA, Goff JP, et al. Neutrophil extracellular trap formation by bovine neutrophils is not inhibited by milk. Vet Immunol Immunopathol 2006;113(1–2):248–55.

31. Buckley CD, Gilroy DW, Serhan CN. Proresolving lipid mediators and mechanisms in the resolution of acute inflammation. Immunity 2014;40(3):315–27.

32. Tabas I, Glass CK. Anti-inflammatory therapy in chronic disease: challenges and opportunities. Science 2013;339(6116):166–72.

33. Bennett M, Gilroy DW. Lipid mediators in inflammation. Microbiol Spectr 2016;4(6). https://doi.org/10.1128/microbiolspec.MCHD-0035-2016.

34. Ricciotti E, FitzGerald GA. Prostaglandins and Inflammation. Arterioscler Thromb Vasc Biol 2011;31(5):986–1000.

35. Raphael W, Halbert L, Contreras GA, et al. Association between polyunsaturated fatty acid-derived oxylipid biosynthesis and leukocyte inflammatory marker expression in periparturient dairy cows. J Dairy Sci 2014;97(6):3615–25.

36. Boutet P, Bureau F, Degand G, et al. Imbalance between lipoxin A4 and leukotriene B4 in chronic mastitis-affected cows. J Dairy Sci 2003;86(11):3430–9.

37. Baldwin CL, Telfer JC. The bovine model for elucidating the role of gammadelta T cells in controlling infectious diseases of importance to cattle and humans. Mol Immunol 2015;66(1):35–47.

38. Sordillo LM. Nutritional strategies to optimize dairy cattle immunity. J Dairy Sci 2016;99(6):4967–82.

39. Sordillo LM, Mavangira V. The nexus between nutrient metabolism, oxidative stress and inflammation in transition cows. Anim Prod Sci 2014;54(9):1204–14.
40. Spears JW, Weiss WP. Role of antioxidants and trace elements in health and immunity of transition dairy cows. Vet J 2008;176(1):70–6.
41. Hogan JS, Weiss WP, Smith KL. Role of vitamin E and selenium in host defense against mastitis. J Dairy Sci 1993;76(9):2795–803.
42. Smith KL, Harrison JH, Hancock DD, et al. Effect of vitamin E and selenium supplementation on incidence of clinical mastitis and duration of clinical symptoms. J Dairy Sci 1984;67(6):1293–300.
43. Canning P, Hassfurther R, TerHune T, et al. Efficacy and clinical safety of pegbovigrastim for preventing naturally occurring clinical mastitis in periparturient primiparous and multiparous cows on US commercial dairies. J Dairy Sci 2017; 100(8):6504–15.
44. Ismail ZB. Mastitis vaccines in dairy cows: Recent developments and recommendations of application. Vet World 2017;10(9):1057–62.
45. Nickerson SC, Sordillo LM. Modulation of the bovine mammary gland. 3rd edition. Champaign (IL): Large Dairy Herd Management; 2017. p. 907–19.

An Update on the Effect of Clinical Mastitis on the Welfare of Dairy Cows and Potential Therapies

Christina S. Petersson-Wolfe, MSc, PhD[a],*,
Kenneth E. Leslie, DVM, MSc[b], Turner H. Swartz, PhD[a]

KEYWORDS

- Mastitis • Animal welfare • Animal behavior • Pain • NSAIDs

KEY POINTS

- Mastitis is a common and economically important disease that compromises the welfare of dairy cows.
- Because cattle are stoic, pain is difficult to quantify in dairy cattle; this stoicism hinders the ability to identify efficacious therapies for pain management to cows with mastitis. However, producers and veterinarians perceive severe clinical mastitis as being very painful.
- Observations of physiologic and behavioral changes should be considered when monitoring for mastitis. Behavioral responses related to pain and discomfort associated with mastitis may include changes in activity, gait, feeding behavior, and self-grooming. Research has consistently identified a decrease in lying time in cows with mastitis relative to healthy cows.
- There is clear benefit to the use of NSAIDs for management of inflammation and alleviation of pain associated with mastitis. Some of the most notable effects include reducing body temperature, restoring rumen activity, and a reduction in pain sensitivity.

INTRODUCTION

Despite the widespread implementation of mastitis control programs, mastitis is the most common and one of the costliest diseases in the dairy industry. Nearly all dairy producers (99.7%) have reported at least one case of mastitis, with clinical mastitis being detected in nearly one-fourth of all cows.[1] Recent reports have estimated the cost of mastitis in Canada at CAD$622 per case[2] and US$326 per case in the United States.[3] This economic burden is caused by treatment costs, discarded milk, and milk

The authors have nothing to disclose.
[a] Department of Dairy Science, Virginia Tech, 175 West Campus Drive, Blacksburg, VA 24061, USA; [b] Department of Population Medicine, University of Guelph, 50 Stone Road East, Guelph, Ontario N1G 2W1, Canada
* Corresponding author.
E-mail address: milk@vt.edu

production losses from potential long-term damage to the mammary gland. Indirect costs from mastitis can include somatic cell count (SCC) penalties or a loss of milk quality premiums and increased culling rate and impaired reproductive performance.[4–6] Collectively, mastitis is a major issue for the dairy industry with broad-ranging impacts and consequences.

Many researchers contend that animals with mastitis have compromised welfare, and are in need of supportive pain management therapy,[7] with some researchers asserting that appropriate analgesic treatment of clinical mastitis, to provide relief from pain, discomfort, and distress, should be mandatory.[8] Recent technological advances have allowed researchers to assess the effects of mastitis on animal behavior and welfare, and the efficacy of mastitis treatments. Several nonsteroidal anti-inflammatory drugs (NSAIDs) are available as supportive therapies for clinical mastitis. This article focuses on recent advances in the assessment, therapy, and effects of mastitis on cow behavior and welfare. This review is an update to "Assessment and Management of Pain in Dairy Cows with Clinical Mastitis."[9]

What Is Sickness Behavior?

Sickness behavior is a term used to describe an evolutionary conserved behavioral adaption used as an all-out attempt to overcome disease.[10,11] Invading pathogens initiate an energy-demanding immune response, such as fever, to increase the effectiveness of the immune system.[12] Consequently, behavioral changes, such as lethargy, anorexia, depression, and a reduction in grooming,[10] occur to enhance the immune response.[12] From an evolutionarily perspective, cattle are considered a prey species, and are inclined to avoid showing pain and vulnerability, even when exposed to harmful stimuli.[13] This stoicism makes identification of sickness behavior, and therefore disease, a challenging task.[14] Recent advances in research have identified behavioral changes associated with disease and discomfort in cattle,[15,16] and are discussed herein.

What Is Pain?

Generally, pain is a subjective term associated with a human experience depending on the individual's experience. The International Association for the Study of Pain defined pain as: "an unpleasant sensory and emotional experience associated with actual or potential tissue damage, or described in terms of such damage."[16] This definition is broad and open to interpretation. Indeed, individuals can construe pain in many different ways, thereby making it extremely difficult to characterize. Although humans can verbally describe their discomfort, we rely on behavioral and physiologic reactions from animals to determine if they are experiencing pain. These responses can differ between species, individual animals, disease stages, and between acute versus chronic conditions. As such, defining pain is a controversial problem. It should be noted that pain behavior and sickness behavior are different; however, in the case of inflammatory disease, such as mastitis, these behavioral changes can converge.

Perception of Pain in Dairy Cattle with Mastitis

Bovine mastitis is an inflammatory disease, typically the result of bacterial infection, and is thought to be painful.[17] Severe clinical cases of mastitis are extremely easy to characterize as being painful.[13] In such cases, the animal shows visible signs of discomfort, including depressed appearance, decreased milk yield, weight loss, abnormal postures, and decreased social interactions.[13] However, mild to moderate cases of mastitis do not present with obvious signs of pain,[13] and the incidence of mild and moderate cases of disease occur at a substantially greater frequency.

Thus, there is considerable potential for a large number of animals to be experiencing pain that may be overlooked. In most cases, it is a lack of understanding of the behavioral changes indicative of animal pain.

In Brazil, a survey was conducted with 124 participating dairy farms, with nearly all farmers (94%) indicating their opinion that cattle do experience pain.[18] A similar pain assessment questionnaire was completed by 149 dairy producers in Norway. This survey evaluated dairy producers' opinions on pain associated with various conditions in dairy cattle using a 0 to 10 scale.[19] Although 70% of surveyed producers did agree that cattle experience pain similarly as humans, there was a wide range of pain scores allocated for the 21 conditions presented, ranging from 2.4 to 8.6. Severe clinical mastitis received a score of 7.6, and moderate clinical mastitis with clots received a score of 5.7. Similarly, a survey of animal health professionals in Scotland indicated that mastitis was not as painful as other clinical conditions or procedures, such as castration, caesarean section, or lameness.[20] However, the greatest variation among respondents was with respect to mastitis. It was concluded that the numerous causative agents involved, the range of environmental conditions, and the varying levels of severity of infection that occur with cases of clinical mastitis may have been responsible for the wide range in response.[20] Another similar survey of veterinarians in the United Kingdom rated severe mastitis at a pain level of 7 (on a 10-point scale) and mild clinical mastitis at a 3.[21] Another study compared the differences in attitudes toward pain between Danish dairy producers and veterinarians.[22] Although dairy farmers and veterinarians agreed that *Escherichia coli* mastitis was the most painful ailment a cow could experience (of 10 ailments listed), there was a discrepancy for mastitis when defined as clots only. Farmers and veterinarians agreed that mastitis (clots only) was considerably less painful than the other ailments; however, farmers rated mastitis as more painful than veterinarians. Altogether, it is evident that several factors about a disease can influence a person's opinion on how much pain an animal is experiencing; however, it does seem that there is a general consensus that severe mastitis is painful in dairy cattle.

Physiologic and Behavioral Indicators Associated with Mastitis in Dairy Cattle

To treat clinical mastitis effectively, it is important to have reliable methods for the detection and classification of severity of infection. The implementation of a clinical evaluation system, which incorporates local and systemic signs of disease, has been found to provide the most sensitive and precise classification system for clinical mastitis, with few false-positive results.[23,24] However, clinical mastitis is still most often detected at milking, by direct observation of the milk and mammary gland. Yet, as farm sizes continue to increase and available labor continues to decrease, dairy producers need to rely more heavily on automated systems, rather than visual detection. Less time is spent on the individual observation of each cow, and there is a greater risk of missing or misdiagnosing a mild or moderate case of clinical mastitis.

Mild and moderate cases of clinical mastitis cases have previously been studied, observing pain thresholds, altered stance, heart rate, respiratory rate, and rectal temperature in affected cows, as compared with control cows.[25–27] Animals with cases of moderate clinical mastitis had higher heart rates, rectal temperatures, and respiratory rates when compared with cows with cases of mild clinical mastitis and normal cows. Cortisol levels and SCC were also significantly higher in cows with mastitis compared with healthy cows.[25] Cows with both mild and moderate mastitis cases had significantly larger hock-to-hock distances compared with normal cows, thereby indicating an altered stance.[26,27] These affected animals also exhibited an increased sensitivity to a mechanical pressure stimulus on the leg closest to the affected mammary quarter, suggesting a change in pain information processing as a result of inflammation. In general, in the case of moderate or mild clinical mastitis, it is more difficult to determine whether dairy cattle experience pain and reduced welfare, as compared with severe cases of mastitis. More recently, in the days before diagnosis of mastitis, cows with mastitis were more restless, indicated by an increase in kicking at milking, and had a reduction in feed intake, and these alterations in behavior persisted after diagnosis as compared with healthy cows.[28] In another study, mastitic cows prior to clinical diagnosis consumed less feed due to a decreased rate of intake (ie, mastitic cows ate slower, less g per min), visited the feeder less, and were less competitive measured by the number of replacements at the feeder.[29] Additionally, cows with mastitis spent less time lying in the days after diagnosis than healthy cows.[28,30] With the difficulties of characterizing a case, and accurately identifying the initiation of illness, in cases of naturally occurring clinical mastitis, models have been developed to induce intramammary inflammation in dairy cattle. In experimentally induced mastitis studies (lipopolysaccharide [LPS] endotoxin or *E coli*), cows with mastitis consumed less feed,[17,31] spent less time eating,[32] reduced rumination or cud chewing,[17,32] reduced self-grooming, spent more time standing idle,[17] spent less time lying,[31–34] and produced less milk.[31] In a *Streptococcus uberis* study, challenged cows were less active, measured in steps per day, for the first 3 days after challenge and produced less milk on d 3, 4, and 5 post-challenge when compared to unchallenged controls.[35] Consistently, these studies have identified an effect of mastitis on lying or standing behaviors. This is particularly concerning because lying is a high-priority behavior that typically increases as part of an adaptive response to overcome disease.[33] One can only speculate as to why mastitis decreases lying time; however, it seems plausible that the increased pressure of an inflamed mammary gland while lying is painful, creating a stimulus to increase standing. Altogether, behavioral and physiologic changes found with severe and moderate clinical mastitis may indicate pain. Therefore, NSAID therapy may be a useful anti-inflammatory, antipyretic, analgesic treatment that could result in improved animal welfare.

THE USE OF NONSTEROIDAL ANTI-INFLAMMATORY DRUGS IN CATTLE

The purpose of anti-inflammatory therapy is to alleviate the pain and other systemic effects that commonly accompany inflammation, and slow any further tissue damage. NSAIDs are commonly used in animals to reduce inflammation (anti-inflammatory), reduce pain (analgesic), reduce pain sensitivity (antihyperalgesic), and decrease overall body temperature (antipyretic). These drugs act mainly by inhibiting cyclooxygenase (COX), which in turn prevents prostaglandin synthesis (**Fig. 1**). NSAIDs are organized into three classes: (1) nonselective (nonspecific), (2) preferential, and (3) selective. The NSAIDs that inhibit COX-1 and COX-2 are referred to as nonselective COX inhibitors, whereas NSAIDs with partial selectively for COX-2 are deemed as COX-2 preferential. Selective COX-2 NSAIDs only inhibit COX-2; however, this type of NSAID is only available in human medicine. In the United States, flunixin meglumine is the only FDA-approved NSAID for use in cattle.[36] Flunixin meglumine is a COX-1 and COX-2 inhibitor, and has greater anti-COX-1 activity than most other NSAIDs.[37] The elimination half-life of flunixin meglumine is 3 to 8 hours,[38] and therefore requires daily dosing.[36] Ketoprofen is another NSAID used by the dairy industry,[39] more so in the European Union and Canada.[36] Ketoprofen inhibits both of the COX pathways and has a short-half-life of 0.42 hours.[40] Carprofen is another NSAID available to dairy producers in the European Union.[36] The chief mode of action of this NSAID is unclear; however, this NSAID does have a long half-life (>37 h).[41] Sodium salicylate is another NSAID available. The half-life

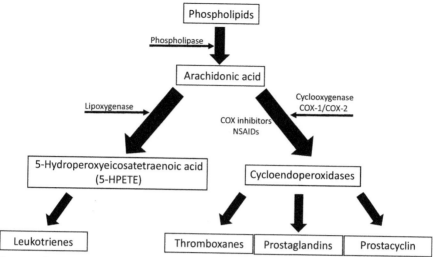

Fig. 1. Inflammatory cascade. Arachidonic acid is converted to cycloendoperoxidases via enzymatic action of cyclooxygenase. Cycloendoperoxidases are converted to prostaglandins, which cause inflammation, pain, and fever. Nonsteroidal anti-inflammatory drugs (NSAIDs) inhibit cyclooxygenase, thereby preventing the synthesis of prostaglandin. (*Adapted from* Summers S. Evidence-based practice part 1: pain definitions, pathophysiologic mechanisms, and theories. J Perianesth Nurs 2000;15:361; with permission.)

of salicylates is short, about 0.5 hours in cattle[42]; however, when administered orally, the elimination half-life can be longer because of the rumen acting as a slow-release reservoir.[36] Sodium salicylate is a weak inhibitor of both COX isoforms,[43] and the more likely mode of action is inhibition of the activation of the proinflammatory transcription factor, nuclear factor kappa-light-chain-enhancer of activated B cells.[44,45] Meloxicam has been approved for use in cattle in many European countries and Canada. Meloxicam is a COX-2 preferential inhibitor in most species[37]; however, this affinity has not been proven in cattle. Meloxicam has an elimination half-life of 23 to 27 hours in low-producing and 17.5 hours in high-producing lactating cattle.[46]

Commercially available NSAIDs are approved for anti-inflammatory and antipyretic indications to relieve clinical signs and promote well-being. NSAIDs are widely used and accepted by veterinarians in dairy practice.[47] Indeed, in a survey of 309 Canadian veterinarians, 93% reported treating acute toxic mastitis cases with analgesia in the form of ketoprofen or flunixin meglumine as supportive therapy.[48] Treatment decisions for animals with severe clinical mastitis most often involve veterinary intervention. Survey research has shown that dairy producers and veterinarians generally agree that severe cases of mastitis can cause the animal significant pain and distress.[48] As such, it is common practice to provide the cow with severe mastitis with NSAID therapy, in addition to antibiotics. Finally, there is mounting evidence for the use of NSAIDs in experimentally induced and naturally occurring models of clinical mastitis, even though formal regulatory approval is rare.

NONSTEROIDAL ANTI-INFLAMMATORY DRUG THERAPY IN CASES OF CLINICAL MASTITIS

In experimental LPS endotoxin models, flunixin meglumine reduced clinical signs of depression,[49] decreased rectal temperature,[49,50] increased rumen motility[50] or cud chewing,[32] increased eating time,[32] and decreased heart rate[50] as compared with nontreated control animals. The administration of ketoprofen reduced rectal temperature, respiration rates, and udder edema, and increased ruminal contractions after LPS challenge.[51] Meloxicam administration after LPS challenge reduced udder edema, body temperature,[52] and pain sensitivity, and increased rumen contractions[53] when compared with control animals. Similarly, intravenous administration of sodium salicylate reduced rectal temperature and concentrations of an inflammatory mediator (prostaglandin $F_{2\alpha}$) in blood during an endotoxin challenge.[54] In an E coli challenge, flunixin meglumine increased dry matter intake and milk production in the days following challenge when compared with challenged control animals.[31] Carprofen administration following E coli challenge reduced rectal temperature and heart rate, and restored reticulorumen motility to prechallenge levels more quickly than untreated control animals.[55]

In cases of mild clinical naturally occurring mastitis, meloxicam therapy in conjunction with an antibiotic reduced the risk of culling, reduced SCC,[56] improved bacteriologic cure rates, and increased reproductive performance when compared with antibiotic therapy alone.[57] In a smaller study, flunixin meglumine administration to acute toxic naturally occurring mastitis reduced rectal temperature at initial examination when compared with control animals; however, no other effect was noted on treatment outcomes.[58] In another flunixin meglumine study, pain sensitivity was assessed using a mechanical device with a blunt pin attached to the hind leg of the cow. The amount of pressure applied determined pain sensitivity. In cows with naturally occurring mastitis, a single treatment of flunixin meglumine reduced pain sensitivity in mild mastitis cases (clots in milk, no visible signs of inflammation in the udder). However, treatment was not effective in cows with moderate cases of mastitis (swollen, hot quarter with clots in milk).[39] Additional doses of flunixin meglumine may be needed for more severe cases of mastitis.[39] In a study in Israel, giving ketoprofen intramuscularly for 5 days allowed affected cows to return to 75% of their daily milk production recorded before their mastitis infection.[59] On initial diagnosis of clinical mastitis, the animals were given antimicrobials in combination with ketoprofen. A secondary portion of the study included ketoprofen-treated animals versus a placebo-treated control group. The animals treated with ketoprofen had an average 93.5% recovery rate based on production parameters as compared with the average recovery rate from the control groups of 78.4%. Furthermore, ketoprofen-treated cows were considerably less likely to be culled that lactation, as only 3% of treated cows were culled, whereas, 22% of untreated control animals were culled.

In general, the use of NSAIDs has been shown to decrease rectal temperatures, decrease signs of inflammation, restore rumen motility, increase eating time and dry matter intake, and reduce heart rates in experimentally induced mastitis cases as compared with their untreated counterparts. Decreased heart rate could be interpreted as a result of a decrease in animal distress or alleviation of pain by the NSAID. There was also an observed reduction in fever of treated animals. Fever is a strategy used by animals to combat infection. As such, it is unknown whether the reduction of fever is actually advantageous for animals with an early case of clinical mastitis. There is generally a lack of published literature supporting the beneficial or detrimental effects of reducing fever in these cases. Although multiple NSAID studies have demonstrated a reduction in clinical signs of inflammation, only a single NSAID study has demonstrated an effect on reducing milk loss after a mastitis challenge.[31] This could potentially be the result of a reduction in inflammation resulting in less damage to the mammary epithelium.

The use of NSAIDs for the treatment of mastitis has been most commonly prescribed for cases of severe endotoxic mastitis, and has not been widely adopted as a standard treatment of cases of mild and moderate clinical mastitis. It is well recognized that for such cases, treatment decisions do not often directly involve veterinarians. Usually, the therapy for these cases at the time of their detection is up to the discretion of the dairy producer or farm manager. Farm personnel often follow a treatment protocol that is designed by farm staff and the herd health advisory team. It is desirable to create a set of standard operating procedures as a treatment protocol for all cases of clinical mastitis and to consult with a veterinarian about how to carry these plans out efficiently. As such, there may be an opportunity for greater use of NSAID therapy in mild and moderate clinical mastitis cases.

FUTURE DIRECTIONS

Because mastitis has long-term detrimental effects on animal welfare, it is key to identify this disease in early stages. Recent research has focused on behavioral observations and assessing physiologic parameters to objectively determine if an animal is experiencing distress caused by a disease. Some of these parameters can be measured on-farm as a tool to identify cows with mastitis. Changes in milk composition, such as SCC, electrical conductivity, L-lactate dehydrogenase, or changes in milk components,[60,61] can all be used as an indicator for mastitis, some of which may be useful in identifying cows with mastitis before clinical signs.[62] Moreover, changes in lying and feeding behaviors before clinical onset of mastitis have been found. For example, a couple days before onset, lying time decreased in cows with mastitis compared with that of healthy cows without mastitis[63]; similarly, feed intake decreased and restless increased (kicking at milking) in the days before clinical mastitis.[28] Taken together, the use of algorithms combining behavioral adaptations to mastitis with changes in milk composition may be useful in identifying cows with mastitis at early stages of disease. This could be particularly useful because pain therapy may be provided at a much earlier stage of disease, which may potentially facilitate a faster recovery with reduced long-term negative consequences.

SUMMARY

It is clear that clinical mastitis has severe detrimental effects on the animal and negative economic impact for dairy producers. However, pain associated with clinical mastitis, generally, is not treated, except in cases of severe acute toxic mastitis. Attention to behavioral and physiologic indicators should be used to monitor animal health. New technologies may allow dairy producers to identify clinical mastitis in its early stages, or even before clinical changes occur. Furthermore, automated measures of lying time show promise as predictors of clinical problems. These new technologies, in addition to other automated measures, have the potential for improving the screening methods for preclinical mastitis, and accurately predicting the onset of a clinical mastitis event. With this opportunity for early detection of infection, there is a potential for early intervention with NSAID therapy, which may allow for maximum efficacy from its use.

Despite which specific NSAID is used, it is clear that the benefits on temperature, rumen function, SCC, milk production, behavior, and pain sensitivity in animals during mastitis indicate that this therapy has a role throughout the dairy industry. To improve animal welfare and reduce long-term negative consequences of mastitis, it is essential that the alleviation of any perceived pain and inflammation associated with clinical mastitis be addressed.

REFERENCES

1. USDA-APHIS. Dairy 2014 milk quality, milking procedures, and mastitis on U.S. Dairies, 2014. Washington, DC: USDA; 2016.

2. Aghamohammadi M, Haine D, Kelton DF, et al. Herd-level mastitis-associated costs on Canadian dairy farms. Front Vet Sci 2018;5:100.

3. Liang D, Arnold LM, Stowe CJ, et al. Estimating US dairy clinical disease costs with a stochastic simulation model. J Dairy Sci 2017;100(2):1472–86.

4. Santos JEP, Cerri RLA, Ballou MA, et al. Effect of timing of first clinical mastitis occurrence on lactational and reproductive performance of Holstein dairy cows. Anim Reprod Sci 2004;80(1):31–45.

5. Barker AR, Schrick FN, Lewis MJ, et al. Influence of clinical mastitis during early lactation on reproductive performance of Jersey cows. J Dairy Sci 1998;81(5):1285–90.

6. Ahmadzadeh A, Frago F, Shafii B, et al. Effect of clinical mastitis and other diseases on reproductive performance of Holstein cows. Anim Reprod Sci 2009; 112(3):273–82.

7. Leslie K, Kielland C, Millman S. Is mastitis painful and is therapy for pain beneficial?. In: National Mastitis Council Annual Meeting Proceedings. Madison (WI). Albuquerque (NM): National Mastitis Council; 2010. p. 114–30.

8. Hillerton J. Mastitis therapy is necessary for animal welfare. International Dairy Federation 1998.

9. Leslie KE, Petersson-Wolfe CS. Assessment and management of pain in dairy cows with clinical mastitis. Vet Clin North Am Food Anim Pract 2012;28(2):289–305.

10. Hart BL. Biological basis of the behavior of sick animals. Neurosci Biobehav Rev 1988;12(2):123–37.

11. Dantzer R, Kelley KW. Twenty years of research on cytokine-induced sickness behavior. Brain Behav Immun 2007;21(2):153–60.

12. Johnson RW. The concept of sickness behavior: a brief chronological account of four key discoveries. Vet Immunol Immunopathol 2002;87(3–4):443–50.

13. Huxley J, Hudson C. Should we control the pain of mastitis? Int Dairy Topics 2007; 6:17–9.

14. Weary DM, Niel L, Flower FC, et al. Identifying and preventing pain in animals. Appl Anim Behav Sci 2006;100(1–2):64–76.

15. Weary DM, Huzzey JM, von Keyserlingk, et al. Board-invited review: using behavior to predict and identify ill health in animals. J Anim Sci 2009;87(2):770–7.

16. (IASP), IAftSoP. Classification of chronic pain, second edition (Revised); 2011. Available at: https://s3.amazonaws.com/rdcms-iasp/files/production/public/Content/ContentFolders/Publications2/ClassificationofChronicPain/Part_III-PainTerms. pdf. Accessed July 2, 2018.

17. Fogsgaard KK, Røntved CM, Sørensen P, et al. Sickness behavior in dairy cows during Escherichia coli mastitis. J Dairy Sci 2012;95(2):630–8.

18. Costa JHC, Hötzel MJ, Longo C, et al. A survey of management practices that influence production and welfare of dairy cattle on family farms in southern Brazil. J Dairy Sci 2013;96(1):307–17.

19. Kielland C, Skjerve E, Østerås O, et al. Dairy farmer attitudes and empathy toward animals are associated with animal welfare indicators. J Dairy Sci 2010; 93(7):2998–3006.

20. Fitzpatrick J, Nolan A, Scott E, et al. Observers' perceptions of pain in cattle. Cattle Pract 2002;10:209–12.

21. Huxley J, Whay H. Current attitudes of cattle practitioners to pain and the use of analgesics in cattle. Vet Rec 2006;159:662–8.

22. Thomsen PT, Anneberg I, Herskin MS. Differences in attitudes of farmers and veterinarians towards pain in dairy cows. Vet J 2012;194(1):94–7.

23. Wenz JR, Barrington GM, Garry FB, et al. Use of systemic disease signs to assess disease severity in dairy cows with acute coliform mastitis. J Am Vet Med Assoc 2001;218(4):567–72.

24. Wenz JR, Garry FB, Barrington GM. Comparison of disease severity scoring systems for dairy cattle with acute coliform mastitis. J Am Vet Med Assoc 2006; 229(2):259–62.

25. Fitzpatrick J, Nolan A, Young F, et al. Objective measurement of pain and inflammation in dairy cows with clinical mastitis. Proceedings of the 9th Symposium of the International Society for Veterinary Epidemiology and Economics. Colorado, USA, 2000.

26. Milne M, Nolan A, Cripps P, et al. Preliminary results of a study on pain assessment in clinical mastitis in dairy cows. In: Proceedings of the International Symposium on Veterinary Epidemiology and Economics. Breckenbridge (CO); 2000. p. 73.

27. Kemp MH, Nolan AM, Cripps PJ, et al. Animal-based measurements of the severity of mastitis in dairy cows. Vet Rec 2008;163(6):175–9.

28. Fogsgaard KK, Bennedsgaard TW, Herskin MS. Behavioral changes in freestall-housed dairy cows with naturally occurring clinical mastitis. J Dairy Sci 2015; 98(3):1730–8.

29. Sepúlveda-Varas P, Proudfoot KL, Weary DM, et al. Changes in behaviour of dairy cows with clinical mastitis. Appl Anim Behav Sci 2016;175:8–13.

30. Medrano-Galarza C, Gibbons J, Wagner S, et al. Behavioral changes in dairy cows with mastitis. J Dairy Sci 2012;95(12):6994–7002.

31. Yeiser EE, Leslie KE, McGilliard ML, et al. The effects of experimentally induced Escherichia coli mastitis and flunixin meglumine administration on activity measures, feed intake, and milk parameters. J Dairy Sci 2012;95(9):4939–49.

32. Zimov JL, Botheras NA, Weiss WP, et al. Associations among behavioral and acute physiologic responses to lipopolysaccharide-induced clinical mastitis in lactating dairy cows. Am J Vet Res 2011;72(5):620–7.

33. Cyples JA, Fitzpatrick CE, Leslie KE, et al. Short communication: The effects of experimentally induced Escherichia coli clinical mastitis on lying behavior of dairy cows. J Dairy Sci 2012;95(5):2571–5.

34. Siivonen J, Taponen S, Hovinen M, et al. Impact of acute clinical mastitis on cow behaviour. Appl Anim Behav Sci 2011;132(3–4):101–6.

35. Kester H, Sorter D, Hogan JS. Activity and milk compositional changes following experimentally induced Streptococcus uberis bovine mastitis. J Dairy Sci 2015; 98(2):999–1004.

36. Coetzee JF. A review of analgesic compounds used in food animals in the United States. Vet Clin North Am Food Anim Pract 2013;29(1):11–28.

37. Beretta C, Garavaglia G, Cavalli M. COX-1 and COX-2 inhibition in horse blood by phenylbutazone, flunixin, carprofen and meloxicam: an in vitro analysis. Pharmacol Res 2005;52(4):302–6.

38. Anderson KL, Neff-Davis CA, Davis LE, et al. Pharmacokinetics of flunixin meglumine in lactating cattle after single and multiple intramuscular and intravenous administrations. Am J Vet Res 1990;51:1464–7.

39. Fitzpatrick JL, Young FJ, Eckersall D, et al. Recognising and controlling pain and inflammation in mastitis. In: Proceedings of the British Mastitis Conference, Institute for Animal Health. Stoneleigh, Coventry. West Midlands (UK); 1998. p. 36–44.

40. Landoni MF, Cunningham FM, Lees P. Pharmacokinetics and pharmacodynamics of ketoprofen in calves applying PK/PD modelling. J Vet Pharmacol Ther 1995; 18(5):315–24.

41. Delatour P, Foot R, Foster A, et al. Pharmacodynamics and chiralpharmacokinetics of carprofen in calves. Br Vet J 1996;152(2):183–98.

42. Kotschwar JL, Coetzee JF, Anderson DE, et al. Analgesic efficacy of sodium sa-licylate in an amphotericin B-induced bovine synovitis-arthritis model. J Dairy Sci 2009;92(8):3731–43.
43. Mitchell JA, Akarasereenont P, Thiemermann C, et al. Selectivity of nonsteroidal antiinflammatory drugs as inhibitors of constitutive and inducible cyclooxyge-nase. Proc Natl Acad Sci U S A 1993;90(24):11693–7.
44. Kopp E, Ghosh S. Inhibition of NF-kappa B by sodium salicylate and aspirin. Sci-ence 1994;265(5174):956–9.
45. Pierce JW, Read MA, Ding H, et al. Salicylates inhibit I kappa B-alpha phosphor-ylation, endothelial-leukocyte adhesion molecule expression, and neutrophil transmigration. J Immunol 1996;156(10):3961–9.
46. EMEA. Scientific discussion, Metacam CVMP/323/97. London, UK; 2007. Available at: http://www.ema.europa.eu/docs/en_GB/document_library/EPAR_-_Scientific_Discussion/veterinary/000033/WC500065773.pdf.
47. Erskine RJ, Wagner S, DeGraves FJ. Mastitis therapy and pharmacology. Vet Clin North Am Food Anim Pract 2003;19(1):109–38.
48. Hewson CJ, Dohoo IR, Lemke KA, et al. Canadian veterinarians' use of analge-sics in cattle, pigs, and horses in 2004 and 2005. Can Vet J 2007;48(2):155–64.
49. Anderson K, Smith A, Shanks R, et al. Efficacy of flunixin meglumine for the treat-ment of endotoxin-induced bovine mastitis. Am J Vet Res 1986;47(6):1366–72.
50. Wagner SA, Apley MD. Effects of two anti-inflammatory drugs on physiologic vari-ables and milk production in cows with endotoxin-induced mastitis. Am J Vet Res 2004;65(1):64–8.
51. Banting A, Banting S, Heinonen K, et al. Efficacy of oral and parenteral ketoprofen in lactating cows with endotoxin-induced acute mastitis. Vet Rec 2008;163(17):506–9.
52. Fitzpatrick CE, Chapinal N, Petersson-Wolfe CS, et al. The effect of meloxicam on pain sensitivity, rumination time, and clinical signs in dairy cows with endotoxin-induced clinical mastitis. J Dairy Sci 2013;96(5):2847–56.
53. Banting A, Schmidt H, Banting S. Efficacy of meloxicam in lactating cows with E. coli endotoxin-induced acute mastitis. J Vet Pharmacol Ther 2000;23(Suppl 1):E4.
54. Morkoç AC, Hurley WL, Whitmore HL, et al. Bovine acute mastitis: effects of intra-venous sodium salicylate on endotoxin-induced intramammary inflammation. J Dairy Sci 1993;76(9):2579–88.
55. Vangroenweghe F, Duchateau L, Boutet P, et al. Effect of carprofen treatment following experimentally induced Escherichia coli mastitis in primiparous cows. J Dairy Sci 2005;88(7):2361–76.
56. McDougall S, Bryan MA, Tiddy RM. Effect of treatment with the nonsteroidal anti-inflammatory meloxicam on milk production, somatic cell count, probability of re-treatment, and culling of dairy cows with mild clinical mastitis. J Dairy Sci 2009;92(9):4421–31.
57. McDougall S, Abbeloos E, Piepers S, et al. Addition of meloxicam to the treatment of clinical mastitis improves subsequent reproductive performance. J Dairy Sci 2016;99(3):2026–42.
58. Dascanio J, Mechor G, Gröhn Y, et al. Effect of phenylbutazone and flunixin me-glumine on acute toxic mastitis in dairy cows. Am J Vet Res 1995;56(9):1213–8.
59. Shpigel N, Chen R, Winkler M, et al. Anti-inflammatory ketoprofen in the treatment of field cases of bovine mastitis. Res Vet Sci 1994;56(1):62–8.
60. Pyörälä S. Indicators of inflammation in the diagnosis of mastitis. Vet Res 2003;34(5):565–78.

61. Kitchen BJ. Bovine mastitis: milk compositional changes and related diagnostic tests. J Dairy Res 1981;48(1):167–88.
62. Hogeveen H, Kamphuis C, Mollenhorst H, et al. Sensors and milk quality: the quest for the perfect alert. Proceedings of the First North American Conference on Precision dairy management. Toronto, Canada, March 2–5, 2010. 2010. p. 138–51.
63. Yeiser EE. The use of activity measures in combination with physiological factors as indicators of disease in dairy cattle. Virginia Tech; 2011.

Moving?

Make sure your subscription moves with you!

To notify us of your new address, find your **Clinics Account Number** (located on your mailing label above your name), and contact customer service at:

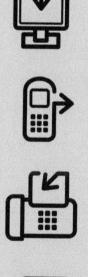

Email: journalscustomerservice-usa@elsevier.com

800-654-2452 (subscribers in the U.S. & Canada)
314-447-8871 (subscribers outside of the U.S. & Canada)

Fax number: 314-447-8029

**Elsevier Health Sciences Division
Subscription Customer Service
3251 Riverport Lane
Maryland Heights, MO 63043**

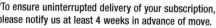

*To ensure uninterrupted delivery of your subscription, please notify us at least 4 weeks in advance of move.

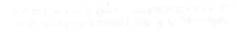

Printed and bound by CPI Group (UK) Ltd, Croydon, CR0 4YY

07/10/2024

01040503-0010